Radiology MCQs

for the new FRCR Part 2A

Shahid Hussain MA MB BChir MRCP
Specialist Registrar Radiology
Royal Orthopaedic Hospital, Birmingham
Sherif Latif MB ChB MRCS
Specialist Registrar Radiology
George Eliot Hospital, Nuneaton
Steve Colley MB ChB MRCS
Specialist Registrar Radiology
Birmingham Children's Hospital
Debbie Tattersall BSc MB ChB MRCP FRCR
Consultant Radiologist
University Hospital Birmingham

tfm Publishing Ltd, Castle Hill Barns, Harley, Nr Shrewsbury, SY5 6LX, UK.
Tel: +44 (0)1952 510061; Fax: +44 (0)1952 510192
E-mail: nikki@tfmpublishing.com; Web site: www.tfmpublishing.com

Design and layout: Nikki Bramhill

ISBN 1 903378 47 8

Printed by Gutenberg Press Ltd., Gudja Road, Tarxien, PLA 19, Malta.

Tel: +356 21897037; Fax: +356 21800069.

Contents

Introduction

This multiple choice book is designed for graduates preparing for the new Fellowship of the Royal College of Radiologists' Part 2A Examination. Having done MCQ exams in radiology and medicine we have found that the best method of preparation for this type of exam, is to attempt as many multiple choice questions as possible, supplementing gaps in knowledge by further reading around the subject and as the exam date approaches, doing practice exams under time constraints to perfect exam technique. This book attempts to provide for these revision methods. The book is divided into two sections. Section 1 contains six chapters mirroring the six modules of the new format exam, in both their subject matter and style of questions.

1. Cardiothoracic and Vascular, including lung, pleura, heart, mediastinum and peripheral vasculature.
2. Musculoskeletal and Trauma, including soft tissues.
3. Gastrointestinal, including liver, biliary, pancreas and spleen.
4. Genitourinary, Adrenal, Obstetrics & Gynaecology and Breast.
5. Paediatrics.
6. Central Nervous System and Head & Neck, including spine, eyes, ENT, salivary glands and dental.

Section 2 contains six practice papers with one complete mock paper for each of the modules.

The questions have been drawn from commonly used radiology textbooks, specialist textbooks and radiology journals, including *Clinical Radiology* and *RadioGraphics*. Therefore, common topics are included, which regularly crop up in exam questions, as well as current up-to-date topics drawn from the journals. These are the sources regularly used by examiners to construct questions. All questions contain brief answers and are fully referenced to allow for further reading.

We hope that we have succeeded in providing a valuable resource to aid in the preparation of the new FRCR Part 2A exam.

Shahid Hussain
Sherif Latif
Steve Colley
Debbie Tattersall
April 2006

Abbreviations

AD	Autosomal dominant
AR	Autosomal recessive
ARDS	Adult respiratory distress syndrome
ASD	Atrial septal defect
CBD	Common bile duct
CNS	Central nervous system
CPPD	Calcium pyrophosphate dihydrate
CSF	Cerebrospinal fluid
CXR	Chest X-ray
DAI	Diffuse axonal injury
DISI	Dorsal intercalated segment instability
DMSA	Dimercaptosuccinic acid
DTPA	Diethylenetriamine penta-acetic acid
FAST	Focused abdominal ultrasonography in trauma
FLAIR	Fluid attenuated inversion recovery
FNH	Follicular nodular hyperplasia
GCT	Giant cell tumour
HIDA	Hepatic 2,6-dimethyl iminodiacetic acid
HPT	Hyperparathyroidism
HRCT	High resolution computed tomography
HU	Hounsfield units
IDA	Iminodiacetic acid
IVC	Inferior vena cava
IVU	Intravenous urography
LOCM	Low osmolar contrast medium
MCPJ	Metacarpophalangeal joint

MDP	Methylene diphosphonate
MEN	Multiple endocrine neoplasms
MIBG	Meta-iodo-benzyl-guanidine imaging
NAI	Non-accidental injury
PDA	Patent ductus arteriosus
PET	Positron emission tomography
PUJ	Pelvi-ureteric junction
SPECT	Single photon emission computed tomography
SVC	Superior vena cava
US	Ultrasound
UTI	Urinary tract infection
VSD	Ventricular septal defect

Acknowledgements

To our families and friends

Section I

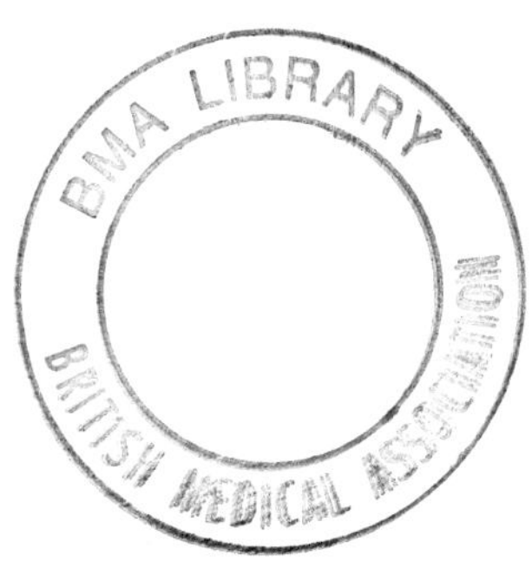

Chapter 1

Cardiothoracic and Vascular

---

1 Chest X-ray appearances of left atrial enlargement include:

a) Splaying of the carina
b) A double shadow of the right heart border
c) Rounding of the apex of the heart
d) Filling in of the concavity of the left heart border above the left main bronchus
e) Displacement of the descending aorta to the left

2 Features of mycotic aneurysms include:

a) Fusiform structure
b) Gradual enhancement with contrast
c) Adjacent vertebral osteomyelitis
d) Adjacent reactive lymph node enlargement
e) Tuberculosis is the commonest infective organism

3 The following are true concerning ultrasound:

a) The frequency of ultrasound used for medical imaging is in the range of 25-40 MHz
b) The velocity of ultrasound waves is proportional to frequency
c) The velocity of sound in soft tissues is 330 metres per second
d) Acoustic impedance is proportional to density
e) At increased frequency there is decreased attenuation of sound waves

4 Buerger's disease (thrombo-angitis obliterans):

a) Is associated with cigarette smoking in 90-95%
b) More commonly affects the upper limb
c) Initially affects the proximal vessels and progresses distally
d) Has multiple corkscrew-shaped collaterals on angiography
e) Has skip lesions as a recognised feature

5 Conditions associated with aortic regurgitation include:

a) Syphilitic aortitis
b) Ankylosing spondylitis
c) Reiter's syndrome
d) Tuberous sclerosis
e) Rheumatoid arthritis

6 Regarding aortic dissection:

a) The Stanford Classification Type B aortic dissection involves the ascending aorta
b) Aortic dissections involving the ascending aorta account for 60-70%
c) Contrast-enhanced CT is more accurate than transoesophageal echocardiography at identifying aortic dissections
d) There is an increased risk in Ehlers-Danlos syndrome
e) Displacement of calcification in the aortic knuckle by >10mm is a useful sign

7 Causes of a large left ventricle include:

a) ASD
b) VSD
c) PDA
d) Thyrotoxicosis
e) Myocarditis

8 Regarding renal artery stenosis:

a) There is an association with neurofibromatosis
b) Fibromuscular dysplasia causes stenosis of the proximal renal artery
c) There is elevation of the renin levels on renal vein sampling of the affected kidney by 50%
d) On IVU, there is early appearance of contrast material in the affected kidney
e) Duplex ultrasound is the investigation of choice

9 The following statements regarding subclavian steal syndrome are true:

a) It is most commonly due to congenital abnormalities
b) On ultrasound there is reversal of contralateral vertebral artery flow
c) Partial steal syndrome is characterised by retrograde flow in systole and antegrade flow in diastole in the vertebral artery
d) There is an association with syphilitic arteritis
e) There are additional lesions of extracranial arteries in 80-90%

10 Concerning carotid artery ultrasound:

a) A low frequency linear probe is used
b) Ultrasound tends to underestimate the degree of stenosis relative to angiography
c) Patients with stenosis of more than 70% of the internal carotid artery are expected to benefit from surgical repair
d) An increase in stenosis of the internal carotid artery is characterised by a reduction in the peak diastolic velocity
e) At the carotid bifurcation, the external carotid artery lies deep to the internal carotid artery

11 The following conditions are associated with atrial septal defects:

a) Turner's syndrome
b) Down's syndrome
c) Klippel-Feil syndrome
d) Noonan syndrome
e) Von Recklinghausen's disease

12 Regarding iodinated intravenous contrast agents:

a) Non-ionic, low osmolar agents are 5-10 times safer than high osmolar ionic agents
b) Patients are advised to remain in the department for at least 15 minutes after the injection
c) There is a specific cross-reactivity between shellfish and low osmolar contrast agents
d) Metformin should be withheld 48 hours before and after intravenous contrast, if serum creatinine is normal in a diabetic patient
e) Breast feeding should be suspended for 7 days following contrast

13 **Features of primary pulmonary hypertension include:**

a) Right descending pulmonary artery more than 25mm wide on plain radiograph
b) Oligaemia
c) Pulmonary artery wider than the aorta on CT images
d) Dilatation of subsegmental vessels on angiography
e) Mosaic attenuation of the lungs on high resolution CT (HRCT)

14 **Causes of oligaemia (decreased pulmonary blood flow) with cyanosis include:**

a) Truncus arteriosus
b) Transposition of great vessels
c) Total anomalous pulmonary venous return
d) Aortic atresia
e) Tetralogy of Fallot

15 **Regarding calcification of the aortic valve:**

a) Bicuspid aortic valve is the commonest cause of aortic valve calcification in patients <30 years of age
b) Rheumatic valve disease is the commonest cause of aortic valve calcification in patients 30-60 years of age
c) Post-stenotic dilatation of the ascending aorta is usually associated with degenerative aortic valve stenosis
d) On a PA chest radiograph the aortic valve lies superior and medial to the pulmonary valve
e) On a lateral chest radiograph the aortic valve lies superior and posterior to the mitral valve

16 **The following are features of cardiac angiosarcoma:**

a) Involves the pericardium in 10-20%
b) Metastasises in 5-10%
c) Most commonly found in the left atrium
d) Usually has a homogenous enhancement pattern on CT
e) Commonly presents in children 3-8 years old

17 The following statements regarding primary cardiac lymphoma are true:

a) It usually affects children 5-10 years of age
b) It is typically of non-Hodgkin's type
c) The right ventricle is the most typical location
d) More than one chamber is affected in less than 5% of patients
e) It presents as a hyperechoic nodule on ultrasound

18 The following structures are enlarged on a PA chest radiograph of a patient with a patent ductus arteriosus:

a) Ascending aorta
b) Aortic arch
c) Left atrium
d) Left ventricle
e) Left pulmonary artery

19 Regarding the pulmonary arteries:

a) The main pulmonary artery is completely confined within the pericardium
b) The right pulmonary artery passes posterior to the superior vena cava
c) The lingula is supplied by the ascending branch of the left pulmonary artey
d) A Judkins-type catheter is commonly used for pulmonary angiography
e) Pulmonary artery pressure of >70mmHg is a relative contraindication to pulmonary angiography

20 Causes of thymic hyperplasia include:

a) Addison's disease
b) Graves' disease
c) Acromegaly
d) Diabetes
e) Post-chemotherapy

21 Fibrosis predominantly affecting the upper lobes is seen in:

a) Rheumatoid arthritis
b) Tuberculosis
c) Bronchopulmonary aspergillosis
d) Sarcoidosis
e) Amiodarone-induced lung fibrosis

22 Regarding anatomy of the diaphragm:

a) The left crus of the diaphragm attaches to the body and discs of L1, L2 and L3 vertebrae
b) The lateral arcuate ligament is a thickening of the fascia over quadratus lumborum
c) The central tendon is fused with the pericardium
d) The inferior vena cava pierces the diaphragm with the right phrenic nerve.
e) Partial reduplication of the diaphragm is commoner on the right side

23 The following are causes of a cavitating lung lesion:

a) Carcinoma of the bronchus
b) Wegener's granulomatosis
c) Rheumatoid nodule
d) Hamartoma
e) Sarcoidosis

24 Regarding Goodpasture's syndrome:

a) Hilar lymph nodes may be enlarged
b) Acute presentation is with air-space consolidation typically at the lung apices
c) Signs of renal failure precede pulmonary complaints
d) Changes are commonly unilateral
e) Prognosis is good

25 The following statements regarding pulmonary hamartomas are correct:

a) 5-10% undergo malignant transformation
b) Calcification is seen in 30-35%
c) 80% are located endobronchially
d) 95% are identified in patients over 40 years
e) Central fat density is identified on CT imaging

26 Regarding pulmonary infections:

a) The characteristic pattern of *Legionella pneumophila* is air space opacification which is initially peripheral
b) Klebsiella pneumonia can present with a bulging interlobar fissure
c) Pseudomonas pneumonia has a predilection for the upper lobes
d) Progressive primary pulmonary tuberculosis is most common in neonates
e) In primary tuberculosis, unilateral pleural effusions are seen in 25% of cases

27 Regarding lymphangioleiomyomatosis:

a) It is found exclusively in females
b) Pulmonary abnormalities are similar to those seen in tuberous sclerosis
c) Cysts commonly have a bizarre outline
d) Cysts show sparing of the apices
e) There is an association with chylothorax

28 Regarding ventilation/perfusion imaging:

a) The 99Tc-DTPA aerosol scan is performed before the perfusion study
b) 81m-Krypton is the cheapest available aerosol for ventilation scanning
c) Severe pulmonary hypertension is a contraindication to ventilation/perfusion scanning
d) Blood should be drawn into the syringe prior to injection of radioisotope for perfusion scanning
e) For the perfusion scan, the patient must remain in position for 15-20 minutes before particles become fixed in the lungs

29 Regarding respiratory CT:

a) HRCT uses 1mm slices at 10-20mm intervals
b) Spatial resolution of HRCT is maximised by using a small field of view
c) 50ml of contrast medium is used for a CT pulmonary angiogram
d) High resolution CT is performed in full expiration
e) CT-guided lung biopsy can be performed as an outpatient with no patient preparation required

30 Causes of ground glass opacity on high resolution CT include:

a) Sarcoidosis
b) Alveolar proteinosis
c) Pulmonary haemorrhage
d) Lymphoma
e) *Pneumocystis carinii* pneumonia

31 Regarding the plain chest radiograph:

a) The lateral radiograph is more sensitive than the erect PA film at detecting pleural fluid
b) A supine view of the chest is most sensitive in detecting pneumothoraces
c) On an erect film an azygous vein of >10mm in diameter is seen in right heart failure
d) The lateral chest radiograph is more sensitive than the erect PA film at detecting free intraperitoneal gas
e) Small pneumothoraces are better visualised on an inspiratory view

32 Causes of eggshell calcification of lymph nodes include:

a) Rheumatoid arthritis
b) Silicosis
c) Histoplasmosis
d) Amyloidosis
e) Scleroderma

33 The following are features of lymphocytic interstitial pneumonitis:

a) Association with Sjögren's syndrome
b) The course in children is more aggressive than in adults
c) Pleural effusions are seen in more than 90%
d) Lymph node enlargement is common
e) Appearance is of bilateral reticulonodular shadowing most pronounced in the mid and lower zones

34 These chest X-ray signs are associated with the following abnormalities:

a) Corona radiata spiculations - primary malignancy
b) Air bronchogram - lymphoma
c) Central calcification - granuloma
d) Decrease in size over time - benign lesion
e) Vessels leading to a mass - rheumatoid nodule

35 Causes of a left-sided pleural effusion include:

a) Rupture of the oesophagus
b) Dissecting aneurysm of the aorta
c) Pancreatitis
d) Gastric neoplasm
e) Transection of the proximal thoracic duct

36 Concerning bronchial adenomas:

a) They can arise in the trachea
b) 80-90% are located centrally in the lung
c) Lesions do not enhance on contrast-enhanced CT
d) Haemoptysis is the presenting feature in 10-15% of patients
e) On CT images, peripheral calcification is seen in 70-80%

37 Squamous cell carcinoma of the lung:

a) Is most often centrally located
b) Has the highest incidence of distant metastases
c) Is the most likely cell type to cause a Pancoast tumour
d) Is the most likely cell type to cause superior venous obstruction
e) Is the commonest lung tumour to cavitate

38 Regarding bronchogenic cysts:

a) Mediastinal bronchogenic cysts account for 85-90%
b) They are associated with spina bifida
c) They may contain air fluid levels
d) Mediastinal bronchogenic cysts are more common on the left
e) Intrapulmonary bronchogenic cysts are found more commonly in the lower lobes

39 The following are features of round pneumonia:

a) More common in adults than children
b) *Haemophilus influenzae* is a causative agent
c) Usually located in the upper lobes
d) Demonstrate a gradual increase in size
e) Posterior location

40 Causes of haemorrhagic lung metastases include:

a) Choriocarcinoma
b) Renal cell carcinoma
c) Melanoma
d) Cervical carcinoma
e) Thyroid carcinoma

41 Features of pulmonary asbestosis include:

a) Increased severity in sub-pleural zones
b) Upper lobe massive fibrosis
c) Hilar adenopathy
d) Thickened interlobular septa on HRCT
e) Increased incidence of bronchio-alveolar cell carcinoma

42 Features of *Pneumocystis carinii* include:

a) Prophylactic use of pentamidine redistributes infection to upper lobes
b) Pleural effusion
c) Hilar lymphadenopathy
d) Pneumatocoeles seen in 10-15% of patients
e) Spontaneous pneumothorax in 30-40%

43 The following statements concerning emphysema are true:

a) Location of the right hemidiaphragm below the anterior aspect of the 6th rib is a sign of overinflation
b) Centrilobular emphysema is related to alpha-1 antitrypsin deficiency
c) Panlobular emphysema is related to cigarette smoking
d) Centrilobular emphysema has a lower lobe predominance
e) Paraseptal emphysema in young adults can present with spontaneous pneumothorax

44 Causes of an apical pleural cap include:

a) Traumatic aortic rupture
b) Pancoast tumour
c) Upper lobe collapse
d) Fibrosing mediastinitis
e) Mediastinal lipomatosis

45 The following pulmonary tumours are benign:

a) Leiomyoma
b) Plasma cell granuloma
c) Askin tumour
d) Kaposi sarcoma
e) Squamous papilloma

46 Features of Wegener's granulomatosis include:

a) Focal glomerulonephritis
b) Migratory polyarthropathy
c) Marked lymphadenopathy
d) Multiple pulmonary nodules with upper lobe predominance
e) Pleural effusion in 3-5%

47 Causes of inferior rib notching include:

a) Coarctation of the aorta
b) Systemic sclerosis
c) Blalock-Taussig shunt
d) Neurofibromatosis Type 1
e) Superior vena caval obstruction

48 Causes of a posterior mediastinal mass include:

a) Aneurysm of the ascending aorta
b) Neuro-enteric cyst
c) Neurofibroma
d) Phaeochromocytoma
e) Teratoma

49 Concerning lymphoma:

a) Hodgkin's disease is more common in the chest than non-Hodgkin's disease
b) Lymph node calcification occurs
c) Posterior mediastinal lymph nodes favour lymphoma rather than sarcoidosis
d) Intrapulmonary lymphoma can present with massive pneumonia-like lobar infiltrates
e) Miliary nodules can be the presenting appearance on chest X-ray

50 The following statements concerning adult respiratory distress syndrome (ARDS) are true:

a) Characteristically, there is a 12-hour delay between clinical onset and chest X-ray abnormalities
b) It is associated with large pleural effusions
c) Pancreatitis is a recognised cause
d) Change is usually unilateral
e) Air bronchograms are more commonly seen in cardiogenic pulmonary oedema than ARDS, allowing differentiation from left heart failure

1 a) True
b) True
c) False - this is a sign of left ventricular enlargement
d) False - this is a feature of enlargement of the infundibulum of the right ventricle. Left atrial enlargement with specific enlargement of the left atrial appendage occurs below the main bronchus
e) True - but rare

Diagnostic Radiology. A Textbook of Medical Imaging. 4th edition. Grainger and Allison. Churchill Livingstone, 2001: 683-7.

2 a) False - saccular
b) False - rapid contrast enhancement
c) True
d) True
e) False - *Staphylococcus aureus.* It is associated with intravenous drug abuse/subacute bacterial endocarditis

Radiology Review Manual. 5th edition. Dahnert. Lippincott, Williams and Wilkins, 2003: 606.

3 a) False - 1-20 MHz
b) False
c) False - 1540 metres per second
d) True
e) False - increased attenuation

Physics for Medical Imaging. Farr, Allisy-Roberts. Bailliere Tindell, 1996: 183-213.

4 a) True
b) False - 80% affect the lower limb
c) False - initially affects the distal vessels and progresses proximally
d) True
e) True

Radiology Review Manual. 5th edition Dahnert. Lippincott, Williams and Wilkins, 2003: 616.

5 a) True
b) True
c) True
d) False
e) True

Radiology Review Manual. 5th edition. Dahnert. Lippincott, Williams and Wilkins, 2003: 610-1.

6 a) False - Type A involves the ascending aorta
b) True
c) False
d) False - in Ehlers-Danlos syndrome there is an increased risk of aneurysms but not dissection
e) True

Diagnostic Radiology. A Textbook of Medical Imaging. 4th edition. Grainger and Allison. Churchill Livingstone, 2001: 956-8.

7 a) False
b) True
c) True
d) True
e) True

Diagnostic Radiology. A Textbook of Medical Imaging. 4th edition. Grainger and Allison. Churchill Livingstone, 2001: 682-9.

8 a) True
b) False - stenosis is seen in the mid and distal renal artery. In atherosclerotic disease, stenosis is seen in the proximal renal artery
c) True
d) False - there is delay due to reduced glomerular filtration rate.
e) False - MRI is the investigation of choice. Ultrasound is inadequate in up to 50%

Radiology Review Manual. 5th edition. Dahnert. Lippincott, Williams and Wilkins, 2003: 947-50.

9 a) False - atherosclerosis accounts for >90%
b) False - reversal of ipsilateral vertebral artery flow
c) True
d) True
e) True

Radiology Review Manual. 5th edition. Dahnert. Lippincott, Williams and Wilkins, 2003: 647-8.

10 a) False - high frequency linear probe
b) False - overestimates degree of stenosis
c) True - some symptomatic patients with 60-70% stenosis may also have some benefit
d) False - an increase in the peak diastolic and systolic velocity
e) False - internal carotid artery lies deep

Sabeti, *et al.* Quantification of Internal Carotid Artery Stenosis with Duplex Ultrasound. *Radiology* 2004; 232: 431-9.

11 a) False
b) True - ostium primum defect
c) True
d) True
e) False

Radiology Review Manual. 5th edition. Dahnert. Lippincott, Williams and Wilkins, 2003: 568-9.

12 a) True
b) True - if high risk then should stay in department for at least 30 minutes after the injection
c) False
d) False - if serum creatinine is elevated then this is the case. If serum creatinine is normal then it should be simply omitted for 48 hours after contrast injection
e) False - only a very small percentage enters the breast milk and almost none is absorbed across the gastrointestinal tract

Standards for Iodinated Intravascular Contrast Agent Administration to Adult Patients. Royal College of Radiologists, July 2005.

13 a) True
b) True
c) True
d) False - there is pruning/tapering of subsegmental vessels
e) True - due to localised variations in lung perfusion

Radiology Review Manual. 5th edition. Dahnert. Lippincott, Williams and Wilkins, 2003: 643-4.

14 a) False - plethora and cyanosis
b) False - plethora and cyanosis
c) False - plethora and cyanosis
d) False - plethora and cyanosis
e) True

Aids to Radiological Differential Diagnosis. 4th edition. Chapman and Nakielny. W.B. Saunders, 2003: 209.

15 a) True
b) True - in patients >65 years of age, aortic valve calcification is due to atherosclerosis in 90%
c) False - associated with bicuspid aortic valve
d) False - inferior and medial to the pulmonary valve, superior to mitral and tricuspid valves
e) False - superior and anterior to the mitral valve

Radiology Review Manual. 5th edition. Dahnert. Lippincott, Williams and Wilkins, 2003: 583-91.

16 a) False - pericardial involvement in 80%
b) False - metastases at presentation in 70-90%
c) False - right atrium
d) False - heterogenous with central necrosis, haemorrhage
e) False - disease of middle-aged men. Rarely seen in children

Araoz, *et al.* CT and MR Imaging of Primary Cardiac Malignancies. *RadioGraphics* 1999; 19: 1421.

17 a) False - mean age is 60 years of age
b) True
c) False - the right atrium is commonest location
d) False - multiple chambers are involved in up to 75% of patients
e) False - hypoechoic

Grebenc, *et al.* Primary Cardiac and Pericardial Neoplasms: Radiologic-Pathologic Correlation. *RadioGraphics* 2000; 20: 1073.

18 a) True
b) True
c) True
d) True
e) True - right ventricle and atrium will also dilate with pulmonary hypertension

Fundamentals of Diagnostic Radiology. 2nd edition. Brant and Helms. Lippincott, Williams and Wilkins, 1999: 532-5.

19 a) True
b) True - posterior to the aorta and superior vena cava
c) False - descending branch supplies lingula and lower lobe
d) False - a pigtail catheter is used. Judkins catheters are used for coronary artery angiography
e) True - other contraindications include left bundle branch block, bleeding abnormalities, right ventricular end-diastolic pressure >20mm Hg and renal insufficiency

Fundamentals of Diagnostic Radiology. 2nd edition. Brant and Helms. Lippincott, Williams and Wilkins, 1999: 609-10.

20 a) True
b) True
c) True
d) False
e) True

Radiology Review Manual. 5th edition. Dahnert. Lippincott, Williams and Wilkins, 2003: 529.

21 a) False - lower lobe
b) True
c) True
d) True
e) False - lower lobe

Aids to Radiological Differential Diagnosis. 4th edition. Chapman and Nakielny. W.B. Saunders, 2003: 151.

22 a) False - the right attaches to L1-L3 and the left attaches to L1 and L2
b) True - the medial arcuate ligament is a thickening of the fascia over the psoas muscle
c) True
d) True - at the level of T8. Oesophagus pierces diaphragm at T10 and aorta, azygous vein and thoracic duct at T12
e) True - this is also known as accessory hemidiaphragm

Anatomy for Diagnostic Imaging. 2nd edition. Ryan, McNichols and Eustace. Saunders, 2004; Chapter 4: 111-3.

23 a) True
b) True
c) True
d) False
e) True

Aids to Radiological Differential Diagnosis. 4th edition. Chapman and Nakielny. W.B. Saunders, 2003: 138-40.

24 a) True - during acute episodes
b) False - the apices are usually spared
c) False - pulmonary features present before renal
d) False - bilateral
e) False - poor prognosis, usually death within 3 years of diagnosis

Fundamentals of Diagnostic Radiology. 2nd edition. Brant and Helms. Lippincott,Williams and Wilkins, 1999: 368.

25 a) False - benign lesions
b) True
c) False - less than 10% are endobronchial. 90% are intrapulmonary and usually within 2cm of the pleura
d) True
e) True

Fundamentals of Diagnostic Radiology. 2nd edition. Brant and Helms. Lippincott, Williams and Wilkins, 1999: 397.
Aids to Differential Diagnosis. 4th edition. Chapman. W.B. Saunders, 2003: 135.

26 a) True
b) True
c) False
d) False - most common in older children/teenagers
e) True

Fundamentals of Diagnostic Radiology. 2nd edition. Brant and Helms. Lippincott, Williams and Wilkins, 1999: Chapter 17.

27 a) True
b) True
c) False - usually uniform round cysts. In Langerhans' cell histiocytosis the cysts have bizarre irregular outlines
d) False - cysts are uniformly distributed. In Langerhans' cell histiocytosis there is sparing of the apices
e) True

Green, *et al.* 'Aunt Minnies' of Thoracic High Resolution CT. *Radiology Now* 2004; 21: 2.

28 a) True
b) False - expensive and limited availability, but does allow for a simultaneous ventilation and perfusion scan
c) True
d) False - this must be avoided to prevent clumping
e) False - the patient must remain in position for 2-3 minutes, then imaged in the sitting position

A Guide to Radiological Procedures. 4th edition. Chapman and Nakielny. W.B. Saunders, 2001: 184-6.

29 a) True
b) True
c) False - 150ml of contrast medium is used
d) False - in full inspiration
e) False - clotting screen is required before the procedure but it can be performed as an outpatient

A Guide to Radiological Procedures. 4th edition. Chapman and Nakielny. W.B. Saunders, 2001: 187-91.

30 a) True
b) True
c) True
d) True
e) True

Aids to Radiological Differential Diagnosis. 4th edition. Chapman and Nakielny. W.B. Saunders, 2003: 171-2.

31 a) True - 50ml of pleural fluid can be seen on the lateral radiograph and 200ml of pleural fluid on the erect film
b) False
c) True - presents as an ovoid deformity above the right main bronchus
d) True - free intraperitoneal gas is seen on 98% of lateral chest radiographs and 80% of erect PA films
e) False - expiratory view

Diagnostic Radiology. A Textbook of Medical Imaging. 4th edition. Grainger and Allison. Churchill Livingstone, 2001: 304-6.

32 a) False
b) True
c) True
d) True
e) True

Diagnostic Radiology. A Textbook of Medical Imaging. 4th edition. Grainger and Allison. Churchill Livingstone, 2001: 512.

33 a) True
b) False - more aggressive in adults
c) False - pleural effusions are seen in 15%
d) False - lymph node enlargement is not seen. If present it should raise the suspicion of lymphoma
e) True

Diagnostic Radiology. A Textbook of Medical Imaging. 4th edition. Grainger and Allison. Churchill Livingstone, 2001: 481.

34 a) True
b) True
c) True - peripheral calcification is associated with malignancy
d) True
e) False - AV malformation

Radiology Review Manual. 5th edition. Dahnert. Lippincott, Williams and Wilkins, 2003: 268-9.

35 a) True
b) True
c) True
d) True
e) False - right-sided effusion

Radiology Review Manual. 5th edition. Dahnert. Lippincott, Williams and Wilkins, 2003: 439.

36 a) True
b) True
c) False - there is marked enhancement
d) False - features in 40-50% of patients
e) False - peripheral calcification is seen in 30-35%

Diagnostic Radiology. A Textbook of Medical Imaging. 4th edition. Grainger and Allison. Churchill Livingstone, 2001: 477.

37 a) True
b) False - lowest
c) True
d) False - small cell carcinoma is the most likely cell type to cause superior venous obstruction
e) True

Radiology Review Manual. 5th edition. Dahnert. Lippincott, Williams and Wilkins, 2003: 467-70.

38 a) True - intrapulmonary bronchogenic cysts account for 15%
b) True
c) True
d) False - more common on the right
e) False - more common in the upper lobes

McAdams, *et al.* Bronchogenic Cyst: Imaging Features with Clinical and Histopathologic Correlation. *Radiology* 2000; 217: 441.

39 a) False
b) True
c) False - usually in the lower lobes
d) False - rapid increase in size
e) True

Radiology Review Manual. 5th edition. Dahnert. Lippincott, Williams and Wilkins, 2003: 522.

40 a) True
b) True
c) True
d) False
e) True

Radiology Review Manual. 5th edition. Dahnert. Lippincott, Williams and Wilkins, 2003: 506.

41 a) True - asbestos fibres have their highest concentrations under the pleura
b) False - lower lobe fibrosis
c) False - no hilar adenopathy
d) True
e) True

Kim, *et al.* Imaging of Occupational Lung Disease. *RadioGraphics* 2001; 21: 1371.

42 a) True
b) False
c) False
d) True
e) False - spontaneous pneumothorax in 5%

Diagnostic Radiology. A Textbook of Medical Imaging. 4th edition. Grainger and Allison. Churchill Livingstone, 2001: 402-3.

43 a) False - 7th rib
b) False - centrilobular emphysema is related to cigarette smoking
c) False - panlobular emphysema is related to alpha-1 antitrypsin deficiency
d) False - centrilobular emphysema has an upper lobe predominance
e) True

Diagnostic Radiology. A Textbook of Medical Imaging. 4th edition. Grainger and Allison. Churchill Livingstone, 2001: 454-5.

44 a) True
b) True
c) True
d) False
e) True

Radiology Review Manual. 5th edition. Dahnert. Lippincott, Williams and Wilkins, 2003: 441.

45
a) True
b) True
c) False
d) False
e) True

Diagnostic Radiology. A Textbook of Medical Imaging. 4th edition. Grainger and Allison. Churchill Livingstone, 2001: 476-9.

46
a) True
b) True
c) False - lymphadenopathy is rare
d) False - multiple pulmonary nodules with lower lobe predominance
e) False - pleural effusion in 25%

Radiology Review Manual. 5th edition. Dahnert. Lippincott, Williams and Wilkins, 2003: 534-5.

47
a) True
b) False
c) True
d) True
e) True

Diagnostic Radiology. A Textbook of Medical Imaging. 4th edition. Grainger and Allison. Churchill Livingstone, 2001: 320.

48
a) False - aneurysm of the descending aorta
b) True
c) True
d) True
e) False - anterior mediastinal mass

Radiology Review Manual. 5th edition. Dahnert. Lippincott, Williams and Wilkins, 2003: 274-6.

49 a) True
b) True - post-radio/chemotherapy
c) False - anterior mediastinal lymph nodes favour lymphoma
d) True
e) True

Radiology Review Manual. 5th edition. Dahnert. Lippincott, Williams and Wilkins, 2003: 502-3.

50 a) True
b) False - no pleural effusion
c) True
d) False - bilateral but asymmetrical
e) False - air bronchograms are more commoner in ARDS

Diagnostic Radiology. A Textbook of Medical Imaging. 4th edition. Grainger and Allison. Churchill Livingstone, 2001: 553-4.

Chapter 2

Musculoskeletal and Trauma

1 Regarding ultrasound of the ankle:

a) Tendons appear as hyperechoic structures
b) Peroneus longus tendon runs anterior to the lateral malleolus
c) The normal Achilles tendon has a flattened crescentic appearance on axial scans
d) The tibialis posterior, flexor digitorum and flexor hallucis longus tendons run posterior to the medial malleolus
e) A high frequency probe is used

2 Concerning metabolic and endocrine arthritides:

a) Gouty tophi are deposits of sodium urate in peri-articular soft tissues
b) Gout is seen more commonly in females
c) Haemochromatosis in the hand commonly affects the 2nd and 3rd metacarpophalangeal joints
d) Alkaptonuria is an autosomal recessive inherited disorder
e) Alkaptonuria most commonly involves the small joints of the hands

3 With regards to the cervical spine:

a) For the erect lateral view of the cervical spine the central beam is directed horizontally to the centre of C3 vertebra
b) The space between the odontoid process and the anterior arch of the atlas (atlanto-dens interval) should not exceed 3mm in adults
c) A Jefferson fracture is unstable
d) A hangman's fracture is usually secondary to a hyperflexion injury
e) A swimmer's view can be used for better demonstration of the C1/C2 junction

4 Concerning dislocations:

a) Anterior dislocation of the hip accounts for 10-20% of all hip dislocations
b) Posterior dislocations of both radius and ulna account for 80-90% of elbow dislocations
c) Anterior dislocation of the shoulder accounts for more then 90% of glenohumeral dislocations
d) A Bankhart lesion is a fracture of the anterior aspect of the superior rim of the glenoid
e) Dislocation of the patella is usually medial

5 Anatomy of the knee joint:

a) The popliteus muscle tendon passes through a portion of the posterior horn of the lateral meniscus
b) The normal medial meniscus is seen as low signal on T1 weighted spin echo and high signal on T2 weighted spin echo MRI images
c) The medial and lateral collateral ligaments are best assessed on sagittal MRI images of the knee
d) The posterior cruciate ligament is attached to the inner aspect of the medial femoral condyle
e) The commonest site of meniscal injury is the posterior horn of the lateral meniscus

6 Causes of 'Bone within Bone' appearance include:

a) Congenital syphilis
b) Infantile cortical hyperostosis
c) Sickle cell disease
d) Oxalosis
e) Paget's disease

7 Features of diaphyseal aclasia (hereditary multiple exostosis) include:

a) Autosomal recessive inheritence
b) Exostoses have a cap of hyaline cartilage, often with a bursa formation over the cap
c) Exostoses arise from the metaphysis and point towards the joint
d) Exostoses stop growing when the nearest epiphyseal centre fuses
e) Malignant transformation to chondrosarcoma occurs in 35-40%

8 Features of Marfan's sydrome include:

a) Pectus excavatum
b) Dural ectasia
c) Disproportionate shortening of the hallux
d) Ligamentous laxity
e) Progressive protrusio acetabuli

9 Desmoid tumours:

a) Are malignant fibrous tumours
b) Are multiple in 40-50% of cases
c) Only rarely occur in the shoulder
d) Are usually of high signal on T1 weighted MRI images
e) Calcify in more than 90%

10 Regarding osteochondritis dissecans:

a) The average age of onset is within the 2nd decade
b) Lesions in the knee are bilateral in 20-30%
c) Lesions in the knee most commonly involve the lateral aspect of the femoral condyle
d) A high signal intensity line around the lesions on T2 weighted MRI images is indicative of instability
e) A grade 2 osteochondritis dissecans lesion is characterised by a displaced fragment

11 Concerning normal anatomical angles:

a) Pes cavus can be diagnosed when the calcaneo-fifth metatarsal angle is <150 degrees
b) A Bohler's angle of <20 degrees suggests a calcaneus fracture
c) The sulcus angle, formed by lines along the condyles on a skyline view of the patella, is 120-125 degrees
d) The normal angle between femoral neck and shaft is <140 degrees in all age groups
e) Coxa vara is associated with a decrease in femoral neck angle

12 Causes of symmetrical periosteal reaction in adults include:

a) Venous insufficiency
b) Hypertrophic osteoarthropathy
c) Thyroid acropachy
d) Fluorosis
e) Phenytoin therapy

13 With regards to radiofrequency ablation:

a) It is used for treatment of osteoid osteoma
b) Ultrasound guidance is the imaging technique of choice
c) Small lesions can be treated with a single electrode
d) It can be performed as a day case
e) It has a role in the palliative treatment of painful vertebral metastases

14 Regarding glomus tumour of bone:

a) Malignant transformation is common
b) It is most commonly found in a subungal location
c) It appears hyperechoic on ultrasound
d) Lesions are of high signal intensity on T1 weighted spin echo images
e) 20-30% of patients present with multiple lesions

15 Malignant fibrous histiocytoma:

a) Is the commonest soft tissue sarcoma in adults >45 years of age
b) Presents as a painless soft tissue mass
c) Rarely calcifies
d) Is most commonly found in a retroperitoneal location
e) Angiomatoid malignant fibrous histiocytoma is frequently seen in <20-year-olds

16 Regarding myositis ossificans:

a) 10-20% of lesions undergo malignant transformation
b) In the acute stages lesions undergo no contrast enhancement on MRI
c) On a plain radiograph lesions are seen to be in contact with the periosteum
d) It affects the large muscles of the extremities in 80-90% of cases
e) Burns are a recognised predisposing factor

17 Telangiectatic osteosarcoma is:

a) The commonest type of osteosarcoma
b) Painless
c) Highly aggressive
d) Low intensity signal on T2 weighted MRI
e) Most commonly found in patients 60-80 years of age

18 Regarding eosinophilic granuloma:

a) Lesions in proximal long bones are usually diaphyseal
b) The commonest site is the skull
c) On MRI, it appears as a well defined lesion of low signal intensity on T1
d) Lesions rarely elicit a periosteal reaction
e) It is a recognised cause of 'floating teeth' appearance

19 Imaging features of the arthropathy of haemochromatosis include:

a) Generalised osteoporosis
b) Most commonly seen in males over 40 years of age
c) Bilateral symmetrical arthropathy
d) Chondrocalcinosis is seen in up to 30% of patients
e) Subchondral cysts

20 Regarding pathology of the knee:

a) Anterior cruciate ligament tears are associated with >70% of Segond fractures
b) Bone bruises are evident on plain radiographs following trauma
c) Meniscal cysts are well defined high signal intensity lesions on T2 weighted MRI
d) Discoid menisci are less prone to meniscal tears
e) Blount disease is characterised by deformity of the lateral tibial epiphysis

21 Regarding carpal injuries:

a) Fractures through the proximal pole of the scaphoid account for 15-20% of scaphoid fractures
b) Scaphoid fractures involving the distal pole have a high incidence of non-union and osteonecrosis
c) Osteonecrosis most frequently becomes apparent 3-4 weeks after injury
d) Triquetral bone fractures are best demonstrated on the AP film
e) In dorsal intercalated segment instability (DISI) the scapholunate angle is less than 30 degrees

22 Fractures:

a) Rolando fracture is an extra-articular comminuted fracture of the base of the 1st metacarpal
b) Calcaneus fractures are bilateral in 5-10%
c) Muscular contraction of the sartorius muscle can result in avulsion of the anteroinferior iliac spine
d) The fracture line in patellar fractures is most commonly longitudinal
e) In adults, clavicle fractures are commonest in the medial third

23 The following conditions can present as multiple sclerotic bone lesions:

a) Osteopoikilosis
b) Mastocytosis
c) Breast metastases following radiotherapy
d) Tuberous sclerosis
e) Sudeck's atrophy

24 The following statements are correct:

a) Paget's disease has a prevalence of 10% in people over the age of 80 years of age
b) Ankylosing spondylitis is found more commonly in Black than Caucasian populations
c) Developmental dysplasia of the hip is more common in males
d) Diffuse idiopathic skeletal hyperostosis commonly presents in children
e) The highest incidence of fibrous dysplasia is between 30-50 years of age

25 The following conditions have a malignant potential:

a) Osteopoikilosis
b) Bone Island
c) Fibrous cortical defect
d) Intra-osseous ganglion
e) Tumoral calcinosis

26 Features of adamantinoma include:

a) Most common presentation in patients >50 years of age
b) Over 90% occur in the tibia
c) Osteosclerotic lesion
d) Lung metastases
e) Avascularity

27 Regarding simple bone cysts:

a) Distal third of the humerus is the commonest site
b) 70% of patients are between 13-18 years of age
c) Usually cause asymmetrical expansion of bone
d) May have a periosteal reaction in the absence of a pathological fracture
e) Recurrence rate after curettage is up to 10%

28 The following are causes of a premature closure of the growth plate:

a) Homocystinuria
b) Sickle cell anaemia
c) Radiotherapy
d) Trauma
e) Juvenile idiopathic arthritis

29 Epidermoid inclusion cysts:

a) Are characterised by a florid lamellar periosteal reaction
b) Commonly calcify
c) Are more commonly found in the right than the left hand
d) When involving the fingers, the terminal phalanx of the ring finger is the most common site
e) Are preceded by a history of trauma

30 Regarding bone metastases:

a) Prostate metastases are always sclerotic
b) Metastases can be excluded in a patient with bone scintigraphy showing no abnormal uptake
c) Metastases located in the medulla are of reduced signal on T1 and increased signal on fat suppressed T2 MRI images
d) Identification of a 'halo' of high signal intensity around a lesion on T2 weighted MRI suggests a benign lesion
e) Melanoma metastases are usually lytic

31 Primary lymphoma of bone:

a) Usually involves the epiphyses
b) Pelvis is involved in >50%
c) Invasion of the soft tissues occurs early
d) Response to radiotherapy is good
e) Predominantly sclerotic tumour is found in 60-70%

32 Radiographical centering points for the following X-rays are correct:

a) PA view of the hand - 4th MCPJ
b) Lateral view of the elbow - lateral epicondyle
c) AP view of the shoulder - coracoid process
d) AP view of the knee - 2.5cm above the lower pole of the patella
e) Lateral view of the ankle - medial malleolus

33 The following statements regarding seronegative arthritides are correct:

a) Ankylosing spondylitis and inflammatory bowel disease typically cause bilateral symmetrical sacroiliac joint disease
b) Large joint involvement in psoriatic arthropathy is common
c) Reiter's syndrome more commonly involves the feet than the hands
d) The interphalangeal joint of the great toe is rarely affected in Reiter's syndrome
e) Psoriatic arthropathy is associated with bilateral syndesmophytes

34 Features of an osteoid osteoma:

a) Pain is typically more intense at night
b) Are more common in flat bones than osteoblastoma
c) In the hands, the distal phalanx is the commonest site of involvement
d) Observed most frequently in patients >25 years of age
e) The nidus may contain calcification

35 Regarding Giant Cell Tumour (GCT):

a) In long bones, GCTs are usually located in the metaphysis
b) 70-80% are located in the femur
c) Rarely produces expansion
d) Recurrence of 25-35% of cases
e) Multiple primary GCTs in the same patient are seen in 10-20% of cases

36 Features of periosteal osteosarcoma:
a) This is the second commonest subtype of osteosarcoma
b) Typically involves the diaphyses of long tubular bones
c) Extension of tumour usually involves the medullary cavity
d) Prognosis of this tumour is better than that of parosteal osteosarcoma
e) Commonly, appearances are of a pedunculated lesion

37 Regarding tumoral calcinosis:
a) Autosomal dominant inheritence
b) More common in Caucasians
c) Associated with an elevated parathyroid hormone
d) Most commonly are found in a para-articular location around the knees
e) Low tendency to recur

38 Causes of hypertrophic osteoarthropathy include:
a) Thymoma
b) Bronchogenic carcinoma
c) Binswanger disease
d) Amyloidosis
e) Chronic active hepatitis

39 Synovial sarcoma:
a) Is commonly intra-articular
b) Is typically painless
c) Most commonly involves the knee
d) 30-40% exhibit amorphous calcification
e) Is low signal on T1 and T2 weighted MRI images

40 Skeletal features of thalassaemia major include:
a) Erlenmeyer flask deformity
b) Arthropathy
c) Osteoporosis
d) Narrowing of medullary cavity
e) Premature fusion of epiphysis

41 Endosteal chondrosarcoma:

a) Is the most common primary bone tumour
b) Usually involves the diaphyses
c) Hyperglycaemia is a recognised paraneoplastic syndrome
d) Associated soft tissue mass is uncommon
e) Flocculent chondroid calcification is characteristic

42 Regarding chondromyxoid fibroma:

a) 70% of patients are under 40 years of age
b) Tumour is common in the skull
c) In long tubular bones they are commonly eccentrically situated diaphyseal lesions
d) Calcification is identified in 50-60%
e) Commonly are of high signal intensity on T2 weighted spin echo MRI

43 Concerning Brodie's abscess:

a) *Staphylococcus aureus* is the commonest organism
b) Most common in the elderly
c) Tibial metaphysis is commonest location
d) It is usually associated with dense marginal sclerosis
e) Gives a 'double-line' effect on MRI

44 Regarding hyperparathyroidism (HPT):

a) Brown tumours occur more frequently in secondary HPT
b) Rugger Jersey spine occurs more frequently in primary HPT
c) Chondrocalcinosis is seen in 15-20%
d) Increased incidence of slipped upper femoral epiphysis is associated with HPT
e) A normal bone scan in about 80%

45 Features of neurofibromatosis Type 1:

a) Solitary neurofibromas are most commonly of low attenuation on CT
b) On MRI are of low signal on T1 and high signal on T2
c) Plexiform neurofibromas are pathognomic for von-Recklinghausen's disease
d) In neurofibromatosis Type 1, approximately 50% of neurofibromas undergo malignant transformation
e) The most common skeletal abnormality is rib notching

46 Concerning radionuclide imaging:

a) Radiotherapy is associated with a focal increased uptake of radioisotope
b) A superscan characteristically shows diffuse increased bone and renal uptake of MDP radioisotope
c) In a patient with a known primary cancer and vertebral skeletal hot spot, there is a 50% chance that the hot spot represents metastases
d) A bone scan is useful in the routine staging of multiple myeloma
e) Following a scaphoid fracture it is normal for the bone scan to remain positive for up to 12 months

47 Regarding ultrasound of soft tissue masses:

a) Ganglion cysts show posterior acoustic enhancement
b) Ganglion cysts can communicate with the tendon sheath
c) Superficial masses are best examined with a 9-13 MHz Frequency Linear Transducer
d) Schwannomas can be differentiated from neurofibromas by ultrasound appearances
e) Lipomas commonly have increased vascularity

48 Features of sarcoid bone involvement include:

a) Well defined lytic lesions
b) Vertebrae are usually involved
c) Reticulated trabecular pattern in the distal phalanges
d) Joint involvement in 70-80%
e) Paravertebral soft tissue mass

49 Concerning enchondromas:

a) Most frequent tumour found in the small bones of the hands
b) In the hands, diaphyses is the most common site
c) Calcification is rare
d) MRI appearances are of low signal on T1 and high signal on T2 spin echo images
e) Maffuci syndrome is characterised by multiple enchondromas and soft tissue cavernous haemangiomas

50 Features of Paget's disease:

a) Pelvis is most commonly affected
b) Increased density of vertebra - 'ivory vertebra'
c) Thickening of ileopectineal line
d) Candle flame lysis
e) Sarcomatous transformation in 10-15%

1 a) True
b) False - posterior
c) True
d) True
e) True

Ultrasound of the Ankle: Anatomy of Tendons, Bursae and Ligaments. *Seminars in MS Radiology* 2005; 9: 3.

2 a) True - gout is characterised by punched out lesions and peri-articular soft tissue tophi. Great toe most commonly affected=podagra
b) False - commoner in males and post-menopausal women
c) True
d) True - deposition of brown-black pigment in the intervertebral disks and articular cartilage
e) False

Orthopaedic Radiology - a Practical Approach. 2nd edition. Greenspan. Raven Press, 1992; Chapter 14.

3 a) False - C4
b) True - <3mm in adults, <5mm in children
c) True - caused by a blow to vertex of the head while in a neutral position. Fracture of anterior and posterior arches of C1
d) False - hyperextension injury resulting in bilateral fractures of the pedicles of C2. Unstable injury. Accounts for 4-7% of all spinal fractures
e) False - for visualisation of C7/C8/T1

Orthopaedic Radiology - a Practical Approach. 2nd edition. Greenspan. Raven Press, 1992; Chapter 10.

4 a) True - lies medial and inferior to acetabulum on pelvis X-ray
b) True - isolated dislocation of the radial head is rare
c) True - 97% are anterior dislocations. Associated with a Hill-Sachs lesion which is a defect in the posterolateral aspect of the humeral head
d) False - inferior rim
e) False - lateral

Orthopaedic Radiology - a Practical Approach. 2nd edition. Greenspan. Raven Press, 1992; Chapter 5.

5 a) True
b) False - low signal on T1 and T2
c) False - coronal
d) True
e) False - posterior horn of medial meniscus is most commonly injured

Orthopaedic Radiology - a Practical Approach. 2nd edition. Greenspan. Raven Press, 1992; Chapter 8.

6 a) True
b) True
c) True
d) True
e) True - acromegaly and radiation are also causes

Radiology Review Manual. 5th edition. Dahnert. Lippincott, Williams and Wilkins, 2003: 184.

7 a) False - AD, presents at 2-10 years of age
b) True
c) False - arise from metaphysis of long bones near epiphyses and point away from the joint
d) True
e) False - <5%

Radiology Review Manual. 5th edition. Dahnert. Lippincott, Williams and Wilkins, 2003: 132.

8 a) True
b) True
c) False - causes disproportionate lengthening
d) True
e) True - other features include arachnodactyly, tall stature, muscle hypoplasia, osteopaenia, pes planus, kyphoscoliosis

Radiology Review Manual. 5th edition. Dahnert. Lippincott, Williams and Wilkins, 2003: 113.

9 a) False - benign. Presents in <40-year-olds. M:F 1:1
b) False - 10-15%
c) False - common location as are thigh and pelvis
d) False - low signal intensity on T1 and T2 with some intermediate areas on T2 MRI images. Heterogenous echo pattern on US
e) False

Diagnosis of Bone and Joint Disorders. 4th edition. Resnick. W.B. Saunders, 2002: 4162-5.

10 a) True - about 15 years of age
b) True
c) True
d) True
e) False - Grade 4 (displaced fragment/loose body in the joint)
Grade 3 (fragment partially detached)
Grade 2 (defect in cartilage)
Grade 1 (focal softening/fissuring)

Muskuloskeletal Imaging Companion. 1st edition. Thomas H. Berquist. Lippincott, Williams and Wilkins, 2002: 232-5.

11 a) True
b) True
c) False - 140 degrees
d) False - in children angle is 150 degrees at birth. Adults normally 120-135 degrees
e) True

Muskuloskeletal Imaging Companion. 1st edition. Thomas H. Berquist. Lippincott, Williams and Wilkins, 2002.

12 a) True
b) True
c) True
d) True
e) False

Radiology Review Manual. 5th edition. Dahnert. Lippincott, Williams and Wilkins, 2003: 12-3.

13 a) True
b) False - CT guidance is used
c) True - large lesions are treated with cluster electrodes
d) True
e) True

Posteraro, *et al.* Radiofrequency Ablation of Bony Metastatic Disease. *Clinical Radiology* 2004; 59 (9): 804-11.

14 a) False - rare
b) True
c) False - hypoechoic appearance on US
d) False - low signal intensity on T1
e) False

Diagnosis of Bone and Joint Disorders. 4th edition. Resnick. W.B. Saunders, 2002: 4197.

15 a) True
b) True - imaging features of low signal on T1/high signal on T2 with variable contrast enhancement
c) True
d) False - 75% are found in the extremities, lower limb>upper limb
e) True

Diagnosis of Bone and Joint Disorders. 4th edition. Resnick. W.B. Saunders, 2002: 4183-5.

16 a) False - non-neoplastic condition of ossification in muscles. Commoner in adults. M:F 1:1
b) False
c) False - separated from periosteum by lucent zone
d) True
e) True

Diagnosis of Bone and Joint Disorders. 4th edition. Resnick. W.B. Saunders, 2002: 4727-9.

17 a) False
b) False
c) True
d) False - high signal T2. Low signal T1
e) False - 15-35 years of age

Muskuloskeletal Imaging Companion. 1st edition. Thomas H. Berquist. Lippincott, Williams and Wilkins, 2002: 557.

18 a) True
b) True
c) False - increased signal on T1 due to xanthomatous histiocytes
d) False - expansile lytic lesion with periosteal reaction, endosteal scalloping
e) True

Radiology Review Manual. 5th edition. Dahnert. Lippincott, Williams and Wilkins, 2003: 108.

19 a) True
b) True
c) False - asymmetrical
d) True
e) True - other features include osteopaenia, joint space narrowing, subchondral sclerosis. Arthropathy resembles degenerative joint disease + CPPD

Diagnosis of Bone and Joint Disorders. 4th edition. Resnick. W.B. Saunders, 2002: 1658-65.

20 a) True - Segond fracture is an avulsion injury at the insertion of the middle third of the capsular ligament on the upper lateral tibia
b) False - easily detected on MRI
c) True
d) False
e) False - medial tibial epiphysis

Muskuloskeletal Imaging Companion. 1st edition. Thomas H. Berquist. Lippincott, Williams and Wilkins, 2002: Chapter 5.

21 a) True - waist fractures are commonest 80%
b) False - proximal pole
c) False - 3-6 months. Characterised by sclerosis and fragmentation
d) False - lateral film
e) False - the normal scapholunate angle is 30-60 degrees. In DISI it is >60-70 degrees. In VISI it is <30 degrees

Orthopaedic Radiology - a Practical Approach. 2nd edition. Greenspan. Raven Press, 1992; 6.11-6.29.

22 a) False - intra-articular fracture
b) True
c) False - sartorius inserts into anterior superior iliac spine. Rectus femoris inserts into anterior inferior iliac spine
d) False - transverse
e) False - middle third

Orthopaedic Radiology - a Practical Approach. 2nd edition. Greenspan. Raven Press, 1992.

23 a) True
b) True
c) True
d) True
e) False

Aids to Radiological Differential Diagnosis. Chapman and Nakielny. 4th edition. W.B. Saunders, 2003: 14.

24 a) True - unusual in under 40-year-olds
b) False - ratio of 3:1
c) False - much commoner in girls
d) False - usually presents in over 50-year-olds
e) False - the highest incidence of fibrous dysplasia is at 3-15 years of age. 75% are seen below 30 years of age

Radiology Review Manual. 5th edition. Dahnert. Lippincott, Williams and Wilkins, 2003: 2-172.

25 a) False
b) False
c) False
d) False
e) False

Radiology Review Manual. 5th edition. Dahnert. Lippincott, Williams and Wilkins, 2003: 2-172.

26 a) False - 10-50-year-olds
b) True - mostly in the middle third
c) False - osteolytic
d) True - 10% of cases
e) False - prominent vascularity

Diagnostic Radiology. A Textbook of Medical Imaging. 4th edition. Grainger and Allison. Churchill Livingstone, 2001: 1897-8.

27 a) False - proximal third of the humerus is commonest, then proximal third of the femur
b) False - 70% are aged 4-10 years and 90% are <20 years of age
c) False - symmetrical. Aneurysmal bone cysts are eccentric
d) False
e) False - 50%

Radiology Review Manual. 5th edition. Dahnert. Lippincott, Williams and Wilkins, 2003: 161.

28 a) False
b) True
c) True
d) True
e) True

Aids to Radiological Differential Diagnosis. Chapman and Nakielny. 4th edition. W.B. Saunders, 2003: 5.

29 a) False
b) False - no calcification
c) False - left >right
d) False - middle finger
e) True

Radiology Review Manual. 5th edition. Dahnert. Lippincott, Williams and Wilkins, 2003: 43.

30 a) False - in a small percentage the metastases can be entirely lytic
b) False - lesions which outgrow their blood supply appear photopaenic
c) True
d) False - highly specific for metastases
e) True

Diagnostic Radiology. A Textbook of Medical Imaging. 4th edition. Grainger and Allison. Churchill Livingstone, 2001: 1871-75.

31 a) False - diaphysis
b) False - 15%
c) False - relatively late
d) True
e) False - 20%. Increased sclerosis post-therapy

Diagnostic Radiology. A Textbook of Medical Imaging. 4th edition. Grainger and Allison. Churchill Livingstone, 2001: 1893-94.

32 a) False - 3rd MCPJ
b) True
c) True
d) False - 2.5cm below the lower pole of the patella
e) True

A Guide to Radiological Procedures. 4th edition. Chapman and Nakielny. W.B. Saunders, 2001.

33 a) True - psoriatic arthropathy and Reiter's syndrome usually produce an asymmetrical pattern of sacroiliac disease
b) False - small joint rheumatoid-like arthritis
c) True
d) False - commonly affected
e) False - usually unilateral syndesmophytes

Fundamentals of Diagnostic Radiology. 2nd edition. Brant and Helms. Lippincott, Williams and Wilkins, 1999: 1028-32.

34 a) True - relieved by salicylates
b) False - osteoblastoma commoner in flat bones and vertebrae. Osteoid osteoma commoner in long tubular bones. 50-60% in femur/tibia
c) False - rare, found in the proximal phalanges
d) True - some cases are found in very young and elderly. M:F 3:1
e) True - usually is uniformly radiolucent <1cm but can contain calcification

Diagnosis of Bone and Joint Disorders. 4th edition. Resnick. W.B. Saunders, 2002: 3767-86.

35 a) True
b) False - femur 30%, tibia 25%, radius 10%, humerus 6%. Rare in the skull
c) False - expansile osteolytic lesion with cortical thinning
d) False - 40-60%. Usually seen within first 2 years after treatment
e) False - 0.5-5% multiple GCTs may be seen in Paget's disease

Diagnosis of Bone and Joint Disorders. 4th edition. Resnick. W.B. Saunders, 2002: 3939-60.

36 a) False - rare. Seen in 10-20-year-olds
b) True - femur and tibia commonest
c) False - medullary cavity uninvolved. Extension into adjacent soft tissues is common
d) False - worse
e) False - tumour base attaches to cortex over entire extent of tumour

Diagnosis of Bone and Joint Disorders. 4th edition. Resnick. W.B. Saunders, 2002: 3825.

37 a) True - autosomal dominant disorder characterised by nodular juxta-articular calcified soft tissue masses
b) False - commoner in blacks. Onset 1st-2nd decade
c) False - normal calcium, alkaline phosphatase, renal function, parathyroid hormone
d) False - knees are almost never affected. Hips are commonest, then elbows, shoulders, feet
e) False - high recurrence rate

Radiology Review Manual. 5th edition. Dahnert. Lippincott, Williams and Wilkins, 2003: 170.

38 a) True
b) True
c) False
d) True
e) True

Radiology Review Manual. 5th edition. Dahnert. Lippincott, Williams and Wilkins, 2003: 103.

39 a) False
b) False
c) True - also commonly seen in hips, ankles, elbows, feet and hands
d) True
e) False - low T1 and high T2

Radiology Review Manual. 5th edition. Dahnert. Lippincott, Williams and Wilkins, 2003: 163.

40 a) True
b) True - secondary to haemochromatosis and CPPD
c) True
d) False - marrow hyperplasia
e) True - seen in 10%

Radiology Review Manual. 5th edition. Dahnert. Lippincott, Williams and Wilkins, 2003: 165.

41 a) False - 3rd commonest after multiple myeloma and osteosarcoma
b) True
c) True - in 85%
d) False - usual
e) False - this is a characteristic feature of exostotic chondrosarcoma

Radiology Review Manual. 5th edition. Dahnert. Lippincott, Williams and Wilkins, 2003: 56-8.

42 a) True - commonest in 2nd-3rd decade. Slightly more frequent in men than women
b) False - found in long tubular bones. 70% in lower extremity. Rare also in sternum, ribs, spine, facial bones
c) False - metaphyseal
d) False - 13%
e) True

Diagnosis of Bone and Joint Disorders. 4th edition. Resnick. W.B. Saunders, 2002: 3866-70.

43 a) True
b) False - children
c) True
d) True
e) True - high signal intensity of granulation tissue surrounded by low signal - due to marked bone sclerosis

Radiology Review Manual. 5th edition. Dahnert. Lippincott, Williams and Wilkins, 2003: 136.

44 a) False - primary
b) False - secondary
c) True - more frequent in secondary HPT
d) True
e) True

Radiology Review Manual. 5th edition. Dahnert. Lippincott, Williams and Wilkins, 2003: 101.

45 a) True
b) True
c) True
d) False - 5%
e) False - scoliosis is commonest abnormality. Other features include: posterior vertebral scalloping; increase in size of intervertebral foramina; bowing of long bones; pseudoarthrosis; cystic osteolytic lesions; 'ribbon ribs' due to superior and inferior rib notching

Hillier, *et al.* The Soft Tissue Manifestations of Neurofibromatosis Type 1. *Clinical Radiology* 2005; 60(9): 960-7.

46 a) False - the endarteritis associated with radiotherapy treatment reduces uptake of radioisotope
b) False - increased bone but loss of visualisation of the kidneys
c) False - in a patient with a known primary cancer 80% of vertebral hot spots represent metastases
d) False
e) False - a positive bone scan at 12 months represents non-union/avascular necrosis

Radiology Review Manual. 5th edition. Dahnert. Lippincott, Williams and Wilkins, 2003: 1080-3.

47 a) True
b) True
c) True
d) False
e) False

Green, Elias. Sonography of Soft Tissue Masses. *Radiology Now* 2004; 21(2): 12-6.

48 a) True
b) False - unusual
c) True
d) False - rarely involved
e) True

Radiology Review Manual. 5th edition. Dahnert. Lippincott, Williams and Wilkins, 2003: 157.

49 a) True - 40-50% of cases
b) True
c) False - common
d) True
e) True

Diagnosis of Bone and Joint Disorders. 4th edition. Resnick. W.B. Saunders, 2002: 3833-45.

50 a) True - 75%
b) True
c) True
d) True - v-shaped lytic defect in diaphyses of long bones
e) False

Radiology Review Manual. 5th edition. Dahnert. Lippincott, Williams and Wilkins, 2003.

Chapter 3

Gastrointestinal

1 The following statements regarding acute pancreatitis are true:

a) Mumps is a recognised cause
b) Pancreatic oedema is a late sign
c) Pancreatic necrosis demonstrated on CT is associated with a mortality of 5-10%
d) Right-sided pleural effusion is seen in 5%
e) Haemorrhagic pancreatitis is diagnosed by the presence of hypodense areas of 5-20 Hounsfield units on CT

2 Regarding hepatocellular carcinoma:

a) It is the commonest primary visceral malignancy in the world
b) Haemochromatosis is a recognised cause
c) Elevated alpha-fetoprotein is found in 50-60% of cases
d) Has a higher incidence in macronodular than micronodular cirrhosis
e) On MR, hepatoma has a well defined, hypointense capsule on T1 weighted images

3 The following are true of positron emission tomography (PET):

a) Noise is higher than in single-photon emission computed tomography
b) Detectors are made of bismuth germinate
c) Resolution is better than in SPECT
d) The effective dose is much higher than in routine gamma imaging
e) It is reliant on the release of gamma rays

4 Regarding MRI of the liver:

a) Fast spin echo involves a series of 180 degree refocusing pulses after the initial 90 degree pulse
b) Hepatocellular carcinoma is best demonstrated 20-30 seconds after contrast injection on a T1 weighted gadolinium-enhanced image
c) Haemangiomas are of uniform low signal on T1 weighted MRI
d) Dynamic imaging of haemangiomas shows a dense peripheral nodular blush during the arterial phase of liver perfusion
e) Hepatocellular carcinoma is usually hypointense on T2 weighted MRI

5 The following statements regarding pancreatic carcinoma are true:

a) 60-70% of pancreatic carcinomas arise in the tail
b) They are usually hypovascular
c) Calcification is common
d) Contiguous organ invasion is rare
e) On ultrasound appears as a hyperechoic pancreatic mass

6 Regarding pancreatic islet cell tumours:

a) Glucagonoma is the commonest functioning islet cell tumour
b) Insulinoma is found predominantly in the pancreatic body and tail
c) Glucagonoma is a hypervascular tumour
d) Glucagonoma undergoes malignant transformation in 5-10%
e) Multiple insulinomas are associated with MEN Type 1

7 Regarding porcelain gallbladder:

a) It is often symptomless
b) It is rarely associated with gallstones
c) Oral cholecystogram shows a non-functioning gallbladder
d) 60-70% develop carcinoma of the gallbladder
e) Acute pancreatitis is a recognised cause

8 Regarding pancreatic cysts:

a) 70-80% of pancreatic cysts are pseudocysts
b) 10% of patients with autosomal dominant polycystic kidney disease have associated pancreatic cysts
c) Pancreatic pseudocysts can occur in the posterior mediastinum
d) Serous cystadenoma is a common malignant tumour found in children
e) Persistent cysts exceeding 5cm in diameter require drainage

9 The following statements regarding splenic lymphoma are true:

a) The spleen is involved at presentation in 30-40% of patients with non-Hodgkin's lymphoma
b) Focal splenic deposits are usually well defined, round lesions of increased brightness on ultrasound
c) When there is lymphomatous involvement of the spleen, splenomegaly is seen in 70-80%
d) Splenic lymphoma deposits commonly calcify
e) Lymph nodes are seen in the splenic hilum in 50% of patients with Hodgkin's lymphoma

10 The following are features of extrahepatic cholangiocarcinoma:

a) It accounts for 10-15% of all cholangiocarcinomas
b) Is most commonly identified in children under 6 years old
c) Inflammatory bowel disease increases the risk by 2 times
d) Most commonly found in the cystic duct
e) Hypovascular on angiography

11 Features of the MEN II syndrome (Sipple's syndrome) include:

a) Insulinoma
b) Phaeochromocytoma
c) Hyperparathyroidism
d) Medullary carcinoma of the thyroid
e) Pituitary adenoma

12 Liver lesions which appear echogenic on ultrasound include:

a) Lymphoma
b) Cervical cancer metastases
c) Colonic carcinoma metastases
d) Hepatoma
e) Treated breast cancer metastases

13 The following are causes of generalised increase in liver echogenicity on ultrasound:

a) Fatty infiltration
b) Cirrhosis
c) Lymphoma
d) Chronic hepatitis
e) Vacuolar degeneration

14 Regarding Budd-Chiari syndrome:

a) It can be caused by obstruction of the suprahepatic IVC
b) On early CT images, the central liver enhances prominently and the peripheral liver weakly
c) The caudate lobe is markedly atrophic
d) On MRI images 'comma-shaped' intrahepatic collateral vessels are seen
e) A 'spider's web' appearance at hepatic venography is characteristic

15 Features of portal hypertension include:

a) Portal vein diameter of >13mm
b) Splenomegaly
c) Reduction in portal vein velocities to 7-12cm/s
d) Schistosomiasis is a recognised cause
e) Loss of portal venous flow in expiration

16 Features of focal nodular hyperplasia (FNH) include:

a) Hypovascular
b) Necrosis and haemorrhage are common
c) 80-90% of tumours are multiple
d) A strong association with oral contraceptive use
e) 50-70% show reduced activity on technetium sulphur colloid scanning

17 Splenic hamartomas are:

a) Usually associated with hamartomas in other locations
b) The most common primary splenic tumour
c) Of reduced attenuation on unenhanced CT
d) Of heterogenous increased signal intensity on T2 weighted MRI images
e) Associated with Turner's syndrome

18 Features of hydatid disease of the liver include:

a) Raised blood eosinophilia count
b) Left lobe is more commonly affected than the right lobe
c) Rarely calcifies
d) On ultrasound, appearances of a heterogenous mass with daughter cysts
e) Communication with right hepatic duct in 50-60%

19 Epidermoid cysts of the spleen:

a) Are multiple in 80%
b) Are usually <1cm in size
c) Peripheral septations are extremely rare
d) Central calcification is seen in 70-80%
e) Are associated with autosomal dominant polycystic kidney disease

20 The following statements are true:

a) Hepatic veins have no valves
b) Ligamentum teres is the obliterated remnant of the umbilical artery
c) The portal vein is formed by the inferior mesenteric vein and splenic vein
d) Hepatic veins drain to the IVC without an extrahepatic course
e) In the Couinaud system - segment 2 and 4a are divided by the left hepatic vein

21 The following are normal post-liver transplant findings:

a) Right pleural effusion
b) Fluid collection around the falciform ligament
c) Sub-hepatic haematoma
d) Increase in the hepatic artery velocity to 300cm/s
e) Periportal low attenuation collar on CT

22 The following statements regarding hepatoblastoma are true:

a) It is the commonest hepatic tumour in children under 3 years
b) There is an increased incidence in Beckwith-Wiedemann syndrome
c) It frequently metastasises to the lung
d) It is associated with an elevated alpha fetoprotein
e) 20% are multifocal

23 Thickened gastric folds are seen in:

a) Eosinophilic gastroenteritis
b) Uncomplicated coeliac disease
c) Menetrier's disease
d) Systemic sclerosis
e) Crohn's disease

24 Target lesions in the stomach are seen in:

a) Melanoma metastases
b) Ectopic pancreatic tissue
c) Radiation enteritis
d) Neurofibroma
e) Leiomyoma

25 Causes of widening of the retrorectal space include:

a) Crohn's disease
b) Radiotherapy
c) Pelvic lipomatosis
d) Enteric duplication cysts
e) Systemic sclerosis

26 The following are gastrointestinal features of systemic sclerosis:

a) Strictures of the gastro-oesophageal junction
b) Dilated small bowel
c) Thickened small bowel mucosal folds
d) Atonic colon
e) Pseudosacculations on the mesenteric border in the colon

27 The following statements concerning oesophageal carcinoma are true:

a) 90% of cases are squamous cell carcinomas
b) Most commonly located in the upper third of the oesophagous
c) Plummer-Vinson syndrome is a recognised predisposing factor
d) Commonest appearance on double contrast barium swallow is of a large ulcer within a bulging mass
e) It is associated with ulcerative colitis

28 The following are imaging features of Candida oesophagitis on double contrast barium swallow:

a) Granular pattern of mucosal oedema
b) Predilection for the lower third of the oesophagus
c) Discrete horizontally orientated plaque lesions
d) Diffuse shaggy oesophagus in AIDS patients with fulminant disease
e) Strictures

29 The following are causes of multiple nodules in the small bowel:

a) Nodular lymphoid hyperplasia
b) Yersinia enterocolitis
c) Canada-Cronkhite syndrome
d) Coeliac disease
e) Waldenstrom macroglobulinaemia

30 Causes of small bowel strictures include:

a) Amyloidosis
b) Potassium chloride tablets
c) Mastocytosis
d) Radiation enteritis
e) Endometriosis

31 Features of Whipple's disease include:

a) Marked small bowel dilatation
b) Thickening of the small bowel folds
c) Delayed small bowel transit time
d) Migratory arthralgia
e) Pericarditis

32 The following statements regarding Meckel's diverticulum are true:

a) Identification of vitelline artery is pathognomonic
b) Is present in 2-3% of the population
c) Located in the mesenteric border of the ileum
d) In children, small bowel enema is the best investigation to identify it
e) Can present as intussusception in children

33 Complications of coeliac disease include:

a) Ulcerative jejuno-ileitis
b) Hyposplenism
c) Small bowel lymphoma
d) Peptic ulceration
e) Oesophageal squamous cell carcinoma

34 Features of pseudomembranous colitis include:

a) An acute infective colitis due to *Clostridium perfringens* toxin
b) Most commonly affects the transverse colon
c) 'Thumbprinting' is seen on the plain abdominal radiograph
d) Bowel wall thickening is the commonest appearance on non-contrast CT images
e) Ascites is a recognised feature

35 Regarding ischaemic colitis:

a) The right colon is involved in 30% of cases
b) Griffith point is the most commonly affected segment
c) Usually occurs in the first decade of life
d) Barium enema is usually only abnormal in 50-60% of cases
e) Portal vein gas is of little clinical significance

36 Concerning adenomatous polyps of the stomach:

a) They are benign
b) There is an association with Peutz-Jeghers syndrome
c) They are most commonly located in the fundus
d) 80% are smaller than 1cm in diameter
e) They are usually multiple

37 Amyloidosis can cause:

a) Loss of peristalsis of the oesophagus
b) Thickening of the rugae of the antrum of the stomach
c) Jejunisation of the ileum
d) Hepatomegaly
e) Malabsorption

38 Side effects of buscopan include:

a) Bradycardia
b) Urinary retention
c) Acute gastric dilatation
d) Blurred vision
e) Allergic reaction

39 Complications of Crohn's disease include:

a) Cholangiocarcinoma
b) Chronic pancreatitis
c) Cirrhosis
d) Psoas abscess
e) Cholelithiasis

40 Imaging features of intussusception on plain radiograph can include:

a) No abnormality
b) Increased gas in the stomach
c) Loss of the inferior hepatic margin
d) Small bowel obstruction in 50-60%
e) 'Pseudokidney' appearance

41 The following statements regarding the stomach are correct:

a) Mesentero-axial volvulus involves rotation around the line extending from cardia to pylorus
b) Hyperparathyroidism is a cause of gastric ulcers
c) Commonest location of gastric diverticulum is juxtacardia on the posterior wall
d) Rolling hiatus hernia accounts for 99% of hiatus hernias
e) Gastric ulcers above the level of the cardia are usually benign

42 The following statements regarding leiomyoma of the oesophagus are true:

a) It is the commonest benign tumour of the oesophagus
b) It rarely calcifies
c) Ulceration is common
d) It is associated with Allport's syndrome
e) It usually involves mid and lower oesophagus

43 **Causes of smooth oesophageal strictures include:**

a) Scleroderma
b) Epidermolysis bullosa
c) Pemphigus
d) Leiomyosarcoma
e) Lymphoma

44 **The conditions below are associated with strictures in the respective locations:**

a) Tuberculosis - ileocaecal region
b) Crohn's disease - ileocaecal region
c) Schistosomiasis - rectosigmoid junction
d) Amoebiasis - rectosigmoid junction
e) Lymphogranuloma venerum - descending colon

45 **The following conditions cause lesions in the terminal ileum:**

a) Ulcerative colitis
b) Actinomycosis
c) Histoplasmosis
d) Lymphoma
e) Dermatomyositis

46 **Features more in keeping with jejunum than ileum include:**

a) 2.5cm width diameter
b) Thicker valvulae conniventes
c) More numerous Peyer's patches
d) One or two arterial arcades with long branches
e) Thinner walls

47 The following statements regarding large bowel obstruction are true:

a) Nodal non-Hodgkin's lymphoma is a cause
b) Peritoneal carcinomatosis is a recognised cause and is most commonly secondary to uterine cancer
c) Lipoma is a recognised cause
d) Volvulus is commoner in the large bowel than the small bowel
e) Gallstones may cause large bowel obstruction

48 Regarding diverticular disease:

a) Colonic diverticulosis affects 70-80% by 80 years of age
b) 10-25% of individuals with colonic diverticular disease develop diverticulitis
c) Rectosigmoid colon is most commonly affected
d) Fistula formation occurs in 40-50% of cases complicating acute diverticulitis
e) Moderate diverticulitis is present when the bowel wall is thickened >3mm

49 Cause of dysphagia include:

a) Candida oesophagitis
b) Enterogenous cyst
c) Chagas' disease
d) Pseudobulbar palsy
e) Pharyngeal pouch

50 Regarding complications following gastrectomy:

a) Anastomotic leakage is most commonly seen in Billroth II surgery
b) Duodenal stump leakage usually results in abscess formation in the right subhepatic space
c) Acute intra-abdominal haemorrhage has an attenuation value of 100-120 Hounsfield units
d) Acute pancreatitis is a recognised complication
e) Local recurrence of gastric cancer most commonly involves the anastomosis/stump

1 a) True - alcohol and gallstones are commonest
b) False - this is the earliest sign
c) False - there is a mortality of more than 20%
d) False - left-sided
e) False - hyperdense areas of 50-70 Hounsfield units

Textbook of Radiology and Imaging. 7th edition. Sutton. Churchill Livingstone, 2002.
Radiology Review Manual. 5th edition. Dahnert. Lippincott, Williams and Wilkins, 2003: 727-31.

2 a) True
b) True - other causes are cirrhosis, hepatitis, alpha-1 antitrypsin deficiency, Wilson's disease, aflatoxin, thorotrast
c) False - 90%
d) True
e) False - increased signal intensity on a T2 weighted image. Peripheral gadolinium enhancement is seen in about 20%

Radiology Review Manual. 5th edition. Dahnert. Lippincott, Williams and Wilkins, 2003: 713-5.

3 a) False - lower
b) True
c) True
d) False
e) False - positive beta particle emission

Physics for Medical Imaging. Farr, Allisy-Roberts. Bailliere Tindell, 1996: 143-6.

4 a) True
b) True
c) True
d) True - though small haemangiomas have a uniform immediate enhancement pattern of the whole lesion
e) False - increased signal intensity on T2 weighted images and reduced signal on T1

Textbook of Radiology and Imaging. 7th edition. Sutton. Churchill Livingstone, 2002: 1025.

5
a) False - 60-70% in the head, 30% body and 10% in the tail
b) True
c) False - about 2%
d) False - 40% invade oesophagus, stomach, duodenum
e) False - hypoechoic

Textbook of Radiology and Imaging. 7th edition. Sutton. Churchill Livingstone, 2002: 1055.

6
a) False - insulinoma
b) False - glucagonoma. Insulinoma has no predilection for any part
c) True - 90% of glucagonomas are hypervascular. 66% of insulinomas
d) False - insulinoma. 80% glucagonomas undergo malignant transformation. 50% have liver metastases at diagnosis
e) True

Radiology Review Manual. 5th edition. Dahnert. Lippincott, Williams and Wilkins, 2003: 724-6.

7
a) True
b) False - 90%
c) True
d) False - 10-20%
e) False

Radiology Review Manual. 5th edition. Dahnert. Lippincott, Williams and Wilkins, 2003: 732-3.

8
a) True - 25% are true cysts, i.e retention/dermoid/malignant cysts
b) True - in von Hippel-Lindau syndrome pancreatic cysts are present in more than 50%
c) True - most commonly found in the lesser sac but can be found in the inguinal region and mediastinum
d) False - benign tumour of elderly women which has a characteristic sunburst calcified appearance with a central fibrotic scar
e) True - to prevent complications of rupture/infection/haemorrhage

Textbook of Radiology and Imaging. 7th edition. Sutton. Churchill Livingstone, 2002.

9 a) True - slightly higher for Hodgkin's lymphoma
b) False - reduced echogenicity
c) False - 50%
d) True
e) False - uncommon

Textbook of Radiology and Imaging. 7th edition. Sutton. Churchill Livingstone, 2002.

10 a) False - extrahepatic is commoner accounting for 90%
b) False - 50-60-year-olds
c) False - 10 times increased risk. Other predisposing factors include sclerosing cholangitis, Caroli's disease, thorotrast exposure, alpha-1 antitrypsin deficiency and autosomal dominant polycystic kidney disease
d) False - most commonly involves the common bile duct
e) False - hypervascular tumour

Radiology Review Manual. 5th edition. Dahnert. Lippincott, Williams and Wilkins, 2003: 685-7.

11 a) False
b) True
c) True
d) True
e) False

Radiology Review Manual. 5th edition. Dahnert. Lippincott, Williams and Wilkins, 2003: 723.

12 a) False
b) False
c) True
d) True
e) True

Radiology Review Manual. 5th edition. Dahnert. Lippincott, Williams and Wilkins, 2003: 720-1.

13 a) True
b) True
c) False
d) True
e) True

Aids to Radiological Differential Diagnosis. 4th edition. Chapman and Nakielny. W.B. Saunders, 2003: 288.

14 a) True - this is primary obstruction. Secondary obstructions commoner and are due to thrombosis in hepatic veins
b) True - 'flip-flop' pattern. On late images the central liver has washed out and peripherally there is enhancement
c) False - caudate lobe is enlarged
d) True
e) True

Fundamentals of Diagnostic Radiology. 2nd edition. Brant and Helms. Lippincott, Williams and Wilkins, 1999: 674.

15 a) True
b) True
c) True
d) True
e) True

Fundamentals of Diagnostic Radiology. 2nd edition. Brant and Helms. Lippincott, Williams and Wilkins, 1999: 673.
Radiology Review Manual. 5th edition. Dahnert. Lippincott, Williams and Wilkins, 2003: 733-5.

16 a) False - hypervascular
b) False - rare in FNH but common in hepatic adenoma
c) False - solitary
d) False - no association. Hepatic adenoma is associated
e) False - 50-70% normal or increased activity

Fundamentals of Diagnostic Radiology. 2nd edition. Brant and Helms. Lippincott, Williams and Wilkins, 1999: 677.

17 a) True
b) False - rare non-neoplastic lesion
c) True
d) True
e) False - splenic haemangiomas are associated

Radiology Review Manual. 5th edition. Dahnert. Lippincott, Williams and Wilkins, 2003: 738.

18 a) True
b) False - right lobe more than the left. Multiple in 20%
c) False - peripheral calcification in 20-30%. Eggshell calcification in the cyst wall is a rare appearance
d) True
e) True - left hepatic duct in 30%. Common hepatic duct in 10%

Pedrosa, *et al.* Hydatid Disease: Radiologic and Pathologic Features and Complications. *RadioGraphics* 2000; 20: 795.

19 a) False - solitary in 80%
b) False - usually 10cm in size
c) False - found in 85%
d) False - calcification in the wall is seen in 10-20%
e) True

Radiology Review Manual. 5th edition. Dahnert. Lippincott, Williams and Wilkins, 2003: 701.

20 a) True
b) False - left umbilical vein
c) False - superior mesenteric vein and splenic vein
d) True
e) True

Anatomy for Diagnostic Imaging. 2nd edition. Ryan, McNichols and Eustace. Chapter 5: 171-4.

21
a) True
b) True
c) True
d) False - this is a sign of hepatic artery stenosis complicating liver transplant
e) True - periportal oedema seen in 20%

Radiology Review Manual. 5th edition. Dahnert. Lippincott, Williams and Wilkins, 2003: 717-8.

22
a) True
b) True
c) False
d) True
e) True

Radiology Review Manual. 5th edition. Dahnert. Lippincott, Williams and Wilkins, 2003: 713.

23
a) True
b) False
c) True
d) False
e) True

Aids to Radiological Differential Diagnosis. 4th edition. Chapman and Nakielny. W.B. Saunders, 2003: 234-5.

24
a) True
b) True
c) False
d) True
e) True

Aids to Radiological Differential Diagnosis. 4th edition. Chapman and Nakielny. W.B. Saunders, 2003: 238.

25
a) True
b) True
c) True
d) True
e) False

Aids to Radiological Differential Diagnosis. 4th edition. Chapman and Nakielny. W.B. Saunders, 2003: 265.

26
a) False - the gastro-oesophageal junction is widely open with marked reflux
b) True
c) True
d) True
e) False - antimesenteric border. In the small bowel pseudodiverticula are found on the mesenteric side

Aids to Radiological Differential Diagnosis. 4th edition. Chapman and Nakielny. W.B. Saunders, 2003: 610-1.

27
a) True
b) False - 20% in the upper third, 30-40% middle third and 30-40% in lower third
c) True
d) False - polypoid/fungating form is commonest
e) False - predisposing factors include Barrett's oesophagus, alcohol abuse, smoking, coeliac disease, achalasia, tylosis

Fundamentals of Diagnostic Radiology. 2nd edition. Brant and Helms. Lippincott, Williams and Wilkins, 1999: 718-9.

28
a) True
b) False - upper half
c) False - longitudinally orientated
d) True
e) True - rare

Fundamentals of Diagnostic Radiology. 2nd edition. Brant and Helms. Lippincott, Williams and Wilkins, 1999: 714.

29 a) True - multiple 2-4mm nodules
b) True
c) True
d) False
e) True

Aids to Radiological Differential Diagnosis. 4th edition. Chapman and Nakielny. W.B. Saunders, 2003: 250-1.

30 a) False
b) True
c) False
d) True
e) True

Aids to Radiological Differential Diagnosis. 4th edition. Chapman and Nakielny. W.B. Saunders, 2003: 245.

31 a) False
b) True - small bowel appearances of micronodularity, thickening of folds and malabsorption
c) False - normal small bowel transit time
d) True
e) True

Radiology Review Manual. 5th edition. Dahnert. Lippincott, Williams and Wilkins, 2003: 865.

32 a) True
b) True
c) False - antimesenteric border
d) False - radionuclide Tc 99m pertechnetate
e) True

Fundamentals of Diagnostic Radiology. 2nd edition. Brant and Helms. Lippincott, Williams and Wilkins, 1999: 749.

33 a) True
b) True
c) True - coeliac disease is also a risk factor for adenocarcinoma of the small bowel, rectum and stomach
d) False
e) True

Radiology Review Manual. 5th edition. Dahnert. Lippincott, Williams and Wilkins, 2003: 860.

34 a) False - *Clostridium difficile* toxin
b) False - 95% located in rectum
c) True
d) True
e) True - in severe cases, ascites is a recognised feature

Kawamoto, *et al.* Pseudomembranous Colitis: Spectrum of Imaging Findings with Clinical and Pathologic Correlation. *RadioGraphics* 1999; 19: 887.

35 a) True - left colon involved in 45-90%
b) True - Griffith point is the superior mesenteric artery/inferior mesenteric artey junction at the splenic flexure
c) False - >50 years
d) False - 90% abnormal, features of bowel wall thickening, loss of haustrations, thumbprinting
e) False - rare but preterminal sign

Weisner, *et al.* CT of Acute Bowel Ischemia. *Radiology* 2003; 226: 635-50.

36 a) False
b) False - association with Gardner's syndrome
c) False - most commonly located in the antrum
d) False - 80% are larger than 2cm
e) False - usually solitary

Feczko, *et al.* Gastric Polyps: Radiological Evaluation and Clinical Significance. *Radiology* 1985; 155: 581.

37 a) True
b) True
c) True
d) True
e) True

Georgiades, *et al.* Amyloidosis: Review and CT Manifestations. *RadioGraphics* 2004; 24: 405-16.

38 a) False - tachycardia
b) True
c) True
d) True
e) True

A Guide to Radiological Procedures. 4th edition. Chapman and Nakielny. W.B. Saunders, 2001: 53.

39 a) True
b) False
c) True
d) True
e) True

Aids to Radiological Differential Diagnosis. 4th edition. Chapman and Nakielny. W.B. Saunders, 2003: 542-3.

40 a) True
b) False - gas-free abdomen due to excess vomiting
c) True
d) False - seen in 25%
e) False - ultrasound sign

Radiology Review Manual. 5th edition. Dahnert. Lippincott, Williams and Wilkins, 2003: 836.

41 a) False - organo-axial volvulus involves rotation around the line extending from cardia to pylorus. Mesentero-axial volvulus involves rotation around the lesser-greater curve line
b) True
c) True - 75%
d) False - sliding hiatus hernia accounts for 99%
e) False - usually fundal ulcers are malignant. 5% of gastric ulcers are malignant

Radiology Review Manual. 5th edition. Dahnert. Lippincott, Williams and Wilkins, 2003: 743-866.

42 a) True
b) False - it is the only oesophageal tumour that calcifies
c) False
d) True
e) True

Radiology Review Manual. 5th edition. Dahnert. Lippincott, Williams and Wilkins, 2003: 839.

43 a) True
b) True
c) True
d) False
e) False

Aids to Radiological Differential Diagnosis. 4th edition. Chapman and Nakielny. W.B. Saunders, 2003: 229.

44 a) True
b) True
c) True
d) False - descending colon
e) False - rectosigmoid juction

Aids to Radiological Differential Diagnosis. 4th edition. Chapman and Nakielny. W.B. Saunders, 2003: 258-9.

45 a) True
b) True - though rare, it usually affects the caecum
c) True - though rare
d) True
e) False

Aids to Radiological Differential Diagnosis. 4th edition. Chapman and Nakielny. W.B. Saunders, 2003: 254.

46 a) False - ileum is 2.5cm diameter while jejunum is 3-3.5cm
b) True
c) False - fewer but they are larger
d) True - the ileum has 4-5 with shorter arterial arcades
e) False - thicker

Anatomy for Diagnostic Imaging. 2nd edition. Ryan, McNichols and Eustace. W.B. Saunders, 2004: 162.

47 a) True - nodes in the mesentery cause extrinsic compression
b) False - ovarian cancer
c) True - rare
d) True
e) True - usually small bowel but can cause complete block of a pathologically narrowed segment in the colon

Sinha, Verma. Multidetector Row Computed Tomography in Bowel Obstruction. Part 2. Large Bowel Obstruction. *Clinical Radiology* 2005; 60 (10): 1068-75.

48 a) True
b) True
c) True
d) False - 14%
e) True

Buckley, *et al.* Computed Tomography in the Imaging of Colonic Diverticulitis. *Clinical Radiology* 2004; 59 (11): 977-83.

49 a) True
b) True
c) True
d) True
e) True

Aids to Radiological Differential Diagnosis. 4th edition. Chapman and Nakielny. W.B. Saunders, 2003: 223-4.

50 a) False - total gastrectomy
b) True
c) False - 20-40 Hounsfield units
d) True
e) True

Kim, *et al.* Postoperative Anastomotic and Pathologic Findings at CT Following Gastrectomy. *RadioGraphics* 2002; 22: 323-36.

Chapter 4
Genitourinary, Adrenal, Obstetrics & Gynaecology and Breast

1 Regarding percutaneous nephrostomy:

a) It is best to target an upper pole calyx
b) A 5-French drain is adequate for an infected system
c) Ideally the guidewire should be passed into the ureter
d) The tract should be dilated to 2-French larger than that of the drainage catheter
e) A straight Amplatz wire should be used

2 The following are branches of the internal iliac artery:

a) Internal pudendal artery
b) Superior gluteal artery
c) Deep circumflex iliac artery
d) Inferior vesical artery
e) Inferior epigastric artery

3 The following are true of transabdominal ultrasound in early pregnancy:

a) Gestational sac should be visible at 4 weeks
b) Yolk sac is only visible from 7 weeks onwards
c) The earliest ultrasound sign of pregnancy is fundal endometrial thickening
d) Cardiac movement should be identifiable in the foetus at 6.5 weeks
e) Biparietal diameter can be used to predict gestational age from 7 weeks

4 The following cause bladder wall calcification:

a) Transitional cell carcinoma
b) Cytotoxin cystitis
c) Sarcoidosis
d) Osteogenic sarcoma metastases
e) Scleroderma

5 Xanthogranulomatous pyelonephritis:
- a) Is more commonly diffuse than segmental
- b) May be caused by *Proteus mirabilis* infection
- c) Causes reduced size of the affected kidney
- d) Pyuria is associated in less than 50%
- e) Is not usually associated with calculi

6 Ovarian fibroma:
- a) Is bilateral in 40%
- b) Is usually well circumscribed
- c) Patients may have basal cell carcinoma
- d) Is usually hyperechoic on ultrasound
- e) Meigs' syndrome is associated with 50%

7 The following renal calculi are radiopaque:
- a) Cystine
- b) Struvite
- c) Calcium oxalate
- d) Xanthine
- e) Urate

8 Regarding scintigraphy:
- a) Gallium-67 citrate is useful in gynaecological malignancies
- b) 99m technetium DTPA is cleared by tubular secretion
- c) 99m technetium DTPA is the best scintigraphic examination to detect renal cortical scarring
- d) 99m technetium DMSA is used for dynamic renal scintigraphy
- e) 99m technetium pertechnetate is used for micturating cystography

9 Phaeochromocytoma:
- a) Is associated with tuberous sclerosis
- b) Affects the bladder
- c) Is bilateral in 20-40% of cases
- d) Is extra-adrenal in 20-30% of cases
- e) Is associated with gastric haemorrhage

10 The following are true regarding renal anatomy:
a) At the hilum the renal vein lies posterior to the renal artery
b) 5% of people have accessory renal arteries
c) The left renal vein is longer than the right
d) The posterior leaf of the renal fascia is referred to as Gerota's fascia
e) The left renal vein receives the left inferior phrenic vein

11 The following are causes of adrenal calcification:
a) Tuberculosis
b) Phaeochromocytoma
c) Adrenal myelolipoma
d) Histoplasmosis
e) Wolman's disease

12 Buscopan is contraindicated in the following:
a) Pyloric stenosis
b) Myasthenia gravis
c) Angina pectoris
d) Pregnancy
e) Closed angle glaucoma

13 The following cause a striated nephrogram:
a) Medullary sponge kidney
b) Amyloidosis
c) Acute papillary necrosis
d) Adult polycystic disease
e) Acute pyelonephritis

14 The following decrease noise in CT scanning:
a) Zoom enlargement of the display
b) Using a narrower window
c) Increasing slice thickness
d) Decreasing the pitch
e) Decreasing the scan time

15 Concerning anatomy of the lower urinary tract:

a) Bladder rupture with fractures of the pelvis is usually extraperitoneal
b) The point of tear in traumatic bladder rupture is usually at the anterior part of bladder
c) The posterior urethra in the male comprises the prostatic and bulbous urethra
d) In a duplex system the ureter draining the lower moiety is associated with ureterocoele
e) The ureter lies anterior to the testicular artery

16 The following are true concerning testicular tumours:

a) 10% of germ cell tumours are bilateral
b) On ultrasound, seminoma is typically seen as a homogenous hyperechoic lesion
c) Embryonal cell carcinoma is normally homogenous on ultrasound
d) Pancreatic adenocarcinoma can metastasise to the testis
e) In 55-60% of cases, seminoma completely replaces the testicular tissue

17 Leukoplakia:

a) Is most commonly caused by chronic infection
b) Most commonly affects the renal pelvis
c) Is associated with calculi
d) Produces passage of gritty flakes which is pathognomonic
e) Causes filling defects in the ureters

18 Meta-iodo-benzyl-guanidine (MIBG) imaging is used to detect the following:

a) Colonic adenocarcinoma
b) Follicular thyroid carcinoma
c) Carcinoid tumour
d) Phaeochromocytoma
e) Neuroblastoma

19 Concerning intravenous urograms:

a) The paediatric dose of contrast is 2ml per kilogram
b) The use of laxatives has been shown to reduce bowel gas, thereby improving image quality
c) The cephalic vein is the preferred injection site
d) The injection should be given slowly so as to reduce risk of a contrast reaction
e) Patients can eat and drink up to 2 hours before the procedure

20 Concerning renal cell carcinoma:

a) It is bilateral in 10-15% of cases
b) Metastases are present at diagnosis in 40%
c) Stranding densities in the perirenal fat are consistent with tumour spread
d) The staging accuracy of MRI is much better than CT
e) Growth into the renal vein occurs in 5-10%

21 The following are features of prune belly syndrome:

a) Large bladder
b) Medial deviation of the ureters
c) Undescended testes
d) Dilatation of the prostatic utricle
e) Generally a good prognosis

22 Raised alpha-fetoprotein is caused by the following:

a) Twins
b) Encephalocoele
c) Renal agenesis
d) Gastroschisis
e) Omphalocoele

23 Medullary sponge kidney:

a) Is bilateral in 95% of cases
b) Is usually first diagnosed in childhood
c) Is an inherited disorder
d) The kidneys are usually small in size
e) Is associated with transient jaundice

24 Concerning the anatomy of the uterus:

a) In children the uterus and cervix are of equal size
b) The body of the uterus may drain to the inguinal lymph nodes
c) The fundus drains to the para-aortic lymph nodes
d) Just lateral to the cervix, the uterine artery passes below the ureter
e) The subendometrial halo is hypoechoic on ultrasound

25 Krukenberg tumour is caused by:

a) Gastric adenocarcinoma
b) Colonic adenocarcinoma
c) Renal cell carcinoma
d) Pancreatic adenocarcinoma
e) Malignant melanoma

26 The following may cause megaureter:

a) Posterior urethral valves
b) Retroperitoneal fibrosis
c) Beckwith-Wiedemann syndrome
d) Diabetes insipidus
e) Ectopic ureter

27 Concerning congenital uterine anomalies:

a) 75% of women with congenital uterine anomalies have fertility problems
b) They are associated with urinary tract anomalies in 80-90%
c) In uterine didelphys there is duplication of the vagina
d) Bicornuate uterus is the commonest anomaly
e) Vaginal atresia may present with hydronephrosis

28 Adrenal metastases:

a) Are present in a quarter of patients with malignant disease
b) Commonly arise from a breast primary
c) Are hyperintense to liver on T1 weighted images
d) Are hyperintense to liver on T2 weighted images
e) 75% of small adrenal masses in patients with known primary malignancy are metastases

29 Contents of the spermatic cord include:

a) Testicular artery
b) Genital branch of genitofemoral nerve
c) Inferior epigastric artery
d) Cremasteric artery
e) Medial umbilical ligament

30 Uterine fibroid embolisation:

a) Can be used to treat intramural as well as pedunculated fibroids
b) Can be performed immediately after cessation of medical treatment for fibroids
c) Is performed using coils
d) The internal iliac artery should be selectively catheterised using a Cobra catheter
e) Premature menopause may occur

31 The following are true concerning MRI artefacts:

a) Truncation artefact is avoided by decreasing the voxel size
b) Susceptibility artefacts are seen around metal implants
c) Susceptibility artefacts are reduced by using gradient-echo rather than spin-echo sequences
d) Aliasing is reduced by increasing the field of view
e) Aliasing is reduced by using a larger surface coil

32 Regarding pyeloureteritis cystica:

a) It is most commonly seen in young adults
b) The most common causative organism is *Proteus mirabilis*
c) Diabetics are predisposed
d) There is a good response to antibiotic therapy
e) There is a risk of malignancy

33 Concerning MRI of the normal female reproductive organs:

a) The endocervical canal is high signal on T2 weighted images
b) The junctional zone is a layer of myometrial cells with a decreased nuclear cellular ratio
c) The ovaries are well seen on T1 weighted images
d) The uterosacral ligaments are best seen on T2 weighted images
e) The outer myometrium is low signal on T2 weighted images

34 The following cause polyhydramnios:

a) Cystic adenomatoid malformation
b) Posterior urethral valves
c) Twin pregnancy
d) Ventricular septal defect
e) Post-maturity

35 Gallium-67 citrate is taken up by the following:

a) Lymphoma
b) Bronchial carcinoma
c) Normal bone marrow
d) Haemangioma
e) Simple renal cysts

36 The following are seen in Beckwith-Wiedemann syndrome:

a) Omphalocoele
b) Gastrointestinal malrotation
c) Polyhydramnios
d) Microglossia
e) Hepatoblastoma

37 Regarding schistosomiasis:

a) Calcification is the most important single imaging feature
b) The bladder usually has a reduced capacity in the early stages
c) Is endemic in parts of the Eastern Mediterranean
d) In the earliest stage, dilatation of the ureter is confined to the upper third
e) Ureteral calculi are rarely seen

38 The following cause cortical nephrocalcinosis:
a) Renal papillary necrosis
b) Milk-alkali syndrome
c) Chronic glomerulonephritis
d) Chronic transplant rejection
e) Sarcoidosis

39 Concerning MRI of renal masses:
a) The wall of a simple cyst is usually visible
b) Renal cell carcinoma is usually hypointense on T2 weighted images
c) Abscess is usually hyperintense on T2 weighted images
d) Angiomyolipoma is hyperintense on T2 fast spin-echo weighted images
e) Lymphoma is hypointense on T1 weighted images

40 Ultrasound features of a breast carcinoma include:
a) Poorly reflective mass
b) Posterior wall enhancement
c) Heterogenous internal echopattern
d) Ill defined mass
e) Posterior acoustic shadowing

41 Differential diagnoses for a single well defined soft tissue density opacity on mammography include:
a) Cyst
b) Lipoma
c) Papilloma
d) Intramammary lymph node
e) Fibroadenoma

42 The following lesions of the breast have spiculated margins:
a) Breast carcinoma
b) Fat necrosis
c) Radial scar
d) Fibroadenoma
e) Lymphoma

43 Regarding anatomy of the breast:

a) The internal mammary artery contributes 50-60% of the blood supply to the breast
b) Lymph flows bi-directionally via superficial and deep lymphatics of the breast
c) Level 3 axillary lymph nodes lie lateral to the medial border of pectoralis minor
d) The breast is entirely invested by the fascia of the chest wall
e) Cooper's ligaments are normally of high signal on T2 weighted MRI

44 Regarding carcinoma of the male breast:

a) 3-5% occur in men with Klinefelter's syndrome
b) Gynaecomastia is the most significant risk factor
c) Tumour is more commonly found in the right breast
d) 40-60% have enlarged lymph nodes at the time of presentation
e) There is an association with males with increased testosterone levels

45 Renal vein thrombosis:

a) Is more common on the right
b) Is most commonly due to membranous glomerulonephritis
c) Causes a striated nephrogram
d) Causes renal enlargement
e) May be secondary to ovarian vein thrombosis

46 Regarding the investigation of renal artery stenosis:

a) Radionuclide scintigraphy may provide the diagnosis
b) Intrarenal Doppler waveforms may show pulsus tardus
c) Renal - aortic peak systolic ratio is >2.5
d) MR angiography underestimates the degree of stenosis
e) Maximum intensity projections are sufficient to interpret stenotic lesions

47 Features of von Hippel-Lindau disease include:

a) Renal cysts are present in over 50%
b) Renal impairment is common
c) Renal angiomas may be distinguished from renal cell carcinoma by imaging
d) Renal cell carcinomas are usually solitary
e) A cyst with an enhancing nodule is suspicious for malignancy

48 Regarding CT of renal trauma:

a) Renal contusions are hypoattenuating during the nephrographic phase of contrast enhancement
b) Grade 2 lacerations are confined to the renal cortex
c) Evidence of acute arterial bleeding indicates a Grade 3 renal injury
d) The cortical rim sign is usually absent with avulsion of the renal artery
e) Absence of perinephric haematoma is typical of renal artery occlusion

49 Concerning imaging of cervical disorders:

a) Cervical tumours tend to be hyperintense on T2 weighted MR sequences
b) Nabothian cysts are low signal on T1 weighted MR
c) Adenoma malignum is associated with Peutz-Jehgers syndrome
d) Cervical tumour invading the rectal mucosa represents stage 3 disease
e) The vaginal wall is hypointense on T2 weighted MR

50 In renal tract tuberculosis:

a) 25% of patients with pulmonary tuberculosis will develop significant renal tuberculosis
b) Renal calcification is uncommon
c) Papillary irregularity on IVU is a late sign
d) A large, distended bladder is seen
e) Ureteral involvement is due to haematogenous spread

1 a) False - mid + lower pole calyces. This has lower risk of pneumothorax
b) False - 6-French uninfected, 8-French for infected
c) True
d) False - 1-French larger
e) False - J wire to avoid perforation of pelvis

Interventional Radiology, a Survival Guide. 2nd edition. Kessel, Robertson. Elsevier, 2005: 281-4.

2 a) True
b) True
c) False - branch of external iliac artery
d) True
e) False - branch of external iliac artery

Anatomy for Diagnostic Imaging. 2nd edition. Ryan, McNichols and Eustace. W.B. Saunders, 2004: 224-5.

3 a) False - 5 weeks
b) False - from 6 weeks
c) True
d) True
e) False - 12-24 weeks

Aids to Radiological Differential Diagnosis. 4th edition. Chapman and Nakielny. W.B. Saunders, 2003: 492-5.

4 a) True
b) True
c) False
d) True
e) False

Radiology Review Manual. 5th edition. Dahnert. Lippincott, Williams and Wilkins, 2003: 889.

5
a) True
b) True
c) False - globally enlarged
d) False - it is seen in 95%
e) False - centrally obstructing staghorn calculus is seen in 75%

Radiology Review Manual. 5th edition. Dahnert. Lippincott, Williams and Wilkins, 2003: 944-5.

6
a) False - less than 10%
b) True
c) True - it is associated with Gorlin's syndrome
d) False - solid hypoechoic mass mostly
e) False - only 1%. Ovarian fibroma with ascites and pleural effusion

Radiology Review Manual. 5th edition. Dahnert. Lippincott, Williams and Wilkins, 2003: 1049-50.

7
a) True - mildly radiopaque
b) True
c) True
d) False
e) False

Fundamentals of Diagnostic Radiology. 2nd edition. Brant and Helms. Lippincott, Williams and Wilkins, 1999: 794-815.

8
a) False
b) False - glomerular filtration
c) False - 99m technetium DMSA as it is retained in the renal cortex
d) False - static renal scintigraphy
e) True

Fundamentals of Diagnostic Radiology. 2nd edition. Brant and Helms. Lippincott, Williams and Wilkins, 1999: 1293-317.
Radiology Review Manual. 5th edition. Dahnert. Lippincott, Williams and Wilkins, 2003: 1075-117.

9 a) True
b) True - in 1% of cases
c) False - 10%
d) False - 10%
e) True - Carney syndrome; triad of extradrenal phaeochromocytoma, gastric leiomyosarcoma and pulmonary chondromas

Radiology Review Manual. 5th edition. Dahnert. Lippincott, Williams and Wilkins, 2003: 935.
Fundamentals of Diagnostic Radiology. 2nd edition. Brant and Helms. Lippincott, Williams and Wilkins, 1999: 330-2.

10 a) False - anterior
b) False - 15-20%
c) True - it passes anterior to the aorta to reach the inferior vena cava
d) False - Zuckerkandl's fascia. Gerota's fascia is the anterior leaf
e) True

Anatomy for Diagnostic Imaging. 2nd edition. Ryan, McNichols and Eustace. W.B. Saunders, 2004: 189-91.

11 a) True
b) True
c) True - calcification present in 20%
d) True
e) True - rare autosomal recessive lipid disorder associated with enlarged calcified adrenal glands, hepatomegaly and splenomegaly

Fundamentals of Diagnostic Radiology. 2nd edition. Brant and Helms. Lippincott, Williams and Wilkins, 1999: 773-4.

12 a) True
b) True
c) False
d) False
e) True

A Guide to Radiological Procedures. 4th edition. Chapman and Nakielny. W.B. Saunders, 2001: 53-4.

13 a) True - fan-shaped streaks radiating from the papilla to the periphery of the kidney
b) False - causes an increasingly dense nephrogram
c) False - causes an increasingly dense nephrogram
d) False - but seen in infantile polycystic disease due to contrast in dilated tubules
e) True

Aids to Radiological Differential Diagnosis. 4th edition. Chapman and Nakielny. W.B. Saunders, 2003: 337-8.

14 a) False - increases noise
b) False - increases noise as each grey level covers a smaller range of CT numbers
c) True
d) True
e) False

Physics for Medical Imaging. Farr, Allisy-Roberts. Bailliere Tindell, 1996: 109-16.

15 a) True - intraperitoneal rupture may occur when the bladder is full
b) False - at the junction of the loose and fixed peritoneum at the posterior part of the bladder
c) False - prostatic and membranous urethra
d) False - the ureter draining the upper moiety
e) False - posterior

Anatomy for Diagnostic Imaging. 2nd edition. Ryan, McNichols and Eustace. W.B. Saunders, 2004: 227-30.

16 a) True
b) False - homogenous hypoechoic lesion sharply delineated from the normal testicular tissue
c) False - heterogenous. More aggressive than seminoma
d) True
e) False - not in the majority

Fundamentals of Diagnostic Radiology. 2nd edition. Brant and Helms. Lippincott, Williams and Wilkins, 1999: 823-72.

17 a) True
b) False - bladder
c) True - in 25-50%
d) True
e) True

Radiology Review Manual. 5th edition. Dahnert. Lippincott, Williams and Wilkins, 2003: 923.

18 a) False
b) False - medullary thyroid carcinoma
c) True
d) True
e) True

Aids to Radiological Differential Diagnosis. 4th edition. Chapman and Nakielny. W.B. Saunders, 2003: 311.

19 a) False - 1ml per kilogram
b) False - not effective
c) False - flow is retarded in the cephalic vein as it pierces the clavipectoral fascia. The median antecubital vein is preferred
d) False - injection should be rapid to maximise the density of the nephrogram
e) False - should have no food for 5 hours prior to examination

A Guide to Radiological Procedures. 4th edition. Chapman and Nakielny. W.B. Saunders, 2001: 141-3.

20 a) False - 2%
b) True
c) False - usually attributable to oedema or fibrosis from previous inflammation
d) False - they are about equal
e) False - 30%

Fundamentals of Diagnostic Radiology. 2nd edition. Brant and Helms. Lippincott, Williams and Wilkins, 1999: 778-9.

21
a) True
b) False - lateral deviation
c) True
d) True
e) False - there is high mortality

Textbook of Radiology and Imaging. 7th edition. Sutton. Churchill Livingstone, 2002: 929-1017.

22
a) True
b) True
c) True
d) True
e) True

Aids to Radiological Differential Diagnosis. 4th edition. Chapman and Nakielny. W.B. Saunders, 2003: 501.

23
a) False - unilateral in 25%
b) False - young to middle-aged adulthood
c) False - sporadic
d) False - normal sized
e) True - Caroli's disease; saccular cystic dilatation of major intrahepatic bile ducts

Fundamentals of Diagnostic Radiology. 2nd edition. Brant and Helms. Lippincott, Williams and Wilkins, 1999: 785.
Radiology Review Manual. 5th edition. Dahnert. Lippincott, Williams and Wilkins, 2003: 926.

24
a) False - equal size at puberty. The cervix is twice the size of the uterus in children
b) True - via the round ligament
c) True
d) False - passes above the ureter
e) True - analogous to the junctional zone on MRI

Anatomy for Diagnostic Imaging. 2nd edition. Ryan, McNichols and Eustace. W.B. Saunders, 2004: 227-30.

25 a) True
b) True
c) False
d) True
e) False

Radiology Review Manual. 5th edition. Dahnert. Lippincott, Williams and Wilkins, 2003: 1044.

26 a) True
b) True
c) False
d) True
e) True

Radiology Review Manual. 5th edition. Dahnert. Lippincott, Williams and Wilkins, 2003: 886.

27 a) False - 25%
b) False - 20-50%
c) True
d) False - septate uterus
e) True - due to a haematocolpos

Radiology Review Manual. 5th edition. Dahnert. Lippincott, Williams and Wilkins, 2003: 1060-1.

28 a) True
b) True
c) False - hypointense
d) True
e) False - 50% of small adrenal masses are benign adenomas in patients with known primary malignancy

Fundamentals of Diagnostic Radiology. 2nd edition. Brant and Helms. Lippincott, Williams and Wilkins, 1999: 771.

29 a) True
b) True
c) False
d) True - a branch of the inferior epigastric artery
e) False

Anatomy for Diagnostic Imaging. 2nd edition. Ryan, McNichols and Eustace. W.B. Saunders, 2004: 232-4.

30 a) False - should not be used if fibroid is pedunculated due to risk of intra-abdominal sepsis
b) False - delay for 3 months as gonadotrophin-releasing hormone analogues may shrink the uterine arteries, making them extremely difficult to catheterise
c) False - polyvinyl alcohol particles
d) True
e) True - in 2%

Interventional Radiology, a Survival Guide. 2nd edition. Kessel, Robertson. Elsevier, 2005: 206-7.

31 a) True
b) True
c) False - the opposite is true
d) True
e) False - smaller surface coil

Physics for Medical Imaging. Farr, Allisy-Roberts. Bailliere Tindell, 1996: 215-51.

32 a) False - 6th decade
b) False - *Escherichia coli*
c) True
d) False
e) True - increased incidence of transitional cell carcinoma of bladder

Radiology Review Manual. 5th edition. Dahnert. Lippincott, Williams and Wilkins, 2003: 945.

33 a) True
b) False - increased nuclear cellular ratio making it low signal on T2 weighting
c) False - intermediate signal intensity with poor intrinsic contrast
d) False - T1 weighted imaging
e) False - intermediate signal intensity

Anatomy for Diagnostic Imaging. 2nd edition. Ryan, McNichols and Eustace. W.B. Saunders, 2004: 240-2.

34 a) True
b) False - causes oligohydramnios
c) True
d) True
e) False - causes oligohydramnios

Radiology Review Manual. 5th edition. Dahnert. Lippincott, Williams and Wilkins, 2003: 989-90.

35 a) True
b) True
c) True
d) False
e) False

Radiology Review Manual. 5th edition. Dahnert. Lippincott, Williams and Wilkins, 2003: 1075-117.
Fundamentals of Diagnostic Radiology. 2nd edition. Brant and Helms. Lippincott, Williams and Wilkins, 1999: 1293-317.

36 a) True
b) True
c) True - in half of cases
d) False - macroglossia
e) True - there is an increased risk of benign and malignant tumours

Radiology Review Manual. 5th edition. Dahnert. Lippincott, Williams and Wilkins, 2003: 1023-4.

37 a) True - it is very commonly seen in the bladder
b) False - only in advanced disease
c) True
d) False - lower third
e) False - commonly seen

Textbook of Radiology and Imaging. 7th edition. Sutton. Churchill Livingstone, 2002: 929-1017.

38 a) False - causes medullary nephrocalcinosis
b) False - causes medullary nephrocalcinosis
c) True - rarely
d) True
e) False - causes medullary nephrocalcinosis

Aids to Radiological Differential Diagnosis. 4th edition. Chapman and Nakielny. W.B. Saunders, 2003: 313-4.

39 a) False - not visible
b) False - iso to hyperintense
c) True
d) True - due to fat. Also hyperintense on T1 weighted images
e) True - homogenously

Aids to Radiological Differential Diagnosis. 4th edition. Chapman and Nakielny. W.B. Saunders, 2003: 330.

40 a) True
b) False - seen with a simple cyst
c) True
d) True
e) True

Aids to Radiological Differential Diagnosis. 4th edition. Chapman and Nakielny. W.B. Saunders, 2003: 363-73.

41 a) True
b) False
c) True
d) True
e) True

Aids to Radiological Differential Diagnosis. 4th edition. Chapman and Nakielny. W.B. Saunders, 2003: 363-73.

42 a) True
b) True
c) True
d) False
e) False

Fundamentals of Diagnostic Radiology. 2nd edition. Brant and Helms. Lippincott, Williams and Wilkins, 1999: 491-525.

43 a) True - the lateral thoracic artery contributes 30% of the blood supply and some also supplied by the perforating branches of the intercostals arteries
b) False - lymph flows uni-directionally superficial to deep
c) False - level 1 axillary lymph nodes lie lateral to the lateral border of pectoralis minor, level 2 lie behind pectoralis minor and level 3 nodes lie medial to the medial border of pectoralis minor
d) True
e) False - low signal on T2 weighted MRI images

Anatomy for Diagnostic Imaging. 2nd edition. Ryan, McNichols and Eustace. W.B. Saunders, 2004: 307-13.

44 a) True
b) False - risk factors include Klinefelter's syndrome, testicular atrophy, lung disease
c) False - left breast
d) True
e) False - association with males with increased oestrogen levels

Radiology Review Manual. 5th edition. Dahnert. Lippincott, Williams and Wilkins, 2003: 556.

45 a) False - left side is more common
b) True
c) True
d) True
e) True - the left ovarian vein drains into the left renal vein

Kawahima, Sandler, *et al.* CT Evaluation of Renovascular Disease. *RadioGraphics* 2000; 20: 1321-40.

46 a) True - ACE inhibitor scintigraphy
b) True - dampened waveforms are seen with significant stenoses
c) False - >3.5
d) False - MR overestimates stenoses
e) False - source images should be analysed

Soulez, Oliva, *et al.* Imaging of Renovascular Hypertension. *RadioGraphics* 2000; 20: 1355-68.

47 a) True - 50-70%
b) False
c) False
d) False - renal cell carcinomas tend to be multicentric and bilateral
e) True

Tattersall, Moore. Von Hippel-Lindau Disease: MRI of Abdominal Manifestations. *Clinical Radiology* 2002; 57: 85-92.

48 a) True
b) False - cortex, medulla +/- collecting system
c) True
d) False
e) True

Kawashima, Sandler, *et al.* Imaging of Renal Trauma; A Comprehensive Review. *RadioGraphics* 2001; 21: 557-74.

49 a) True
b) False - intermediate to high signal on T1, and high T2 signal
c) True
d) False - stage 4 disease
e) True

Okamoto, Tanaka, *et al.* MR Imaging of the Uterine Cervix. *RadioGraphics* 2003; 23: 425-45.

50 a) False - 4-8%
b) False - common (24-44% of cases)
c) False - an early sign
d) False - reduced bladder capacity
e) False - passage of infected urine

Gibson, Puckett, Shelley. Renal Tuberculosis. *RadioGraphics* 2004; 24: 251-6.

Chapter 5

Paediatrics

1 Which of the following are true of non-accidental injury (NAI):

a) Cerebral injury from shaking is most common over 2 years of age
b) Diaphyseal fractures are more common than metaphyseal fractures
c) Multiple rib fractures are highly suspicious of NAI
d) Interhemispheric subdural haematoma is an atypical finding
e) Spiral fracture of the tibia is highly suspicious

2 Meckel's diverticulum:

a) Is the most common congenital anomaly of the gastrointestinal tract
b) Represents failure of closure of the omphalomesenteric duct
c) Is more common in males
d) Most symptomatic cases arise in childhood
e) Gastrointestinal bleeding is the most common complication

3 Paediatric intussusception:

a) Accounts for over 75% of paediatric intestinal obstruction
b) Typically occurs between 4-8 years of age
c) Plain films are typically abnormal
d) A lead point is identified in over 50% of cases
e) Pneumoperitoneum is a contraindication to air reduction

4 Childhood rhabdomyosarcoma:

a) Is the most common soft tissue sarcoma in children
b) Is the most common pelvic malignant neoplasm in children
c) Genito-urinary tumours account for 25% of cases
d) Orbital tumours are highly malignant
e) T2 weighted MRI is ideal for assessing tumours of prostatic origin

5 Regarding vesico-ureteric reflux:

a) UTI is more common in male neonates
b) Renal scarring is related to the degree of vesico-ureteric reflux
c) Radionuclide imaging may provide the diagnosis
d) Posterior urethral valves represent vestiges of the Wolffian duct
e) Hypertension is a known complication

6 Prune belly syndrome:

a) The bladder is hypoplastic
b) Is associated with abdominal wall deficiency
c) Is accompanied by cryptorchidism in males
d) Ureters are of normal calibre on IVU
e) Pulmonary hypoplasia is a complication

7 Medullary calcification of the kidneys occurs in:

a) Hyperparathyroidism
b) Renal tubular acidosis
c) Pseudohyperparathyroidism
d) Medullary sponge kidney
e) Chronic glomerulonephritis

8 Radiological features of achondroplasia include:

a) Decreased interpedicular distance caudally within the spine
b) Short ribs
c) Dilatation of the lateral cerebral ventricles
d) Anterior vertebral scalloping
e) Relative shortening of the fibula

9 Slipped upper femoral epiphysis:

a) Is seen typically between 4-8 years of age
b) Is bilateral in one third of cases
c) The Line of Klein should intersect the normal femoral head
d) The epiphysis slips posteromedially
e) Subchondral lucency is an early sign

10 The radiological features of pyknodysostosis include:

a) Limb overgrowth
b) Multiple wormian bones
c) Reduced bone density
d) Resorption of the lateral end of the clavicle
e) Tapered distal phalanges

11 Regarding normal skeletal variants:

a) Bipartite patella typically involves the upper outer quadrant
b) The medial humeral epicondyle ossification centre appears after the lateral epicondyle
c) A prominent anterior fat pad indicates intra-articular injury
d) The scaphoid bone is the first carpal bone to ossify
e) Os radiale externum is the commonest supernumary bone around the wrist

12 Multiple wormian bones are a feature of:

a) Rickets
b) Osteogenesis imperfecta
c) Down's syndrome
d) Hypothyroidism
e) Chondrodysplasia punctata

13 The following are CNS features of tuberous sclerosis:

a) Presentation is usually with seizures
b) Subependymal nodules are most common in the occipital horns of the lateral ventricles
c) Cortical tubers are most prominent on T1 weighted MRI
d) Pilocytic astrocytoma is a complication
e) Calcification may be seen in up to 50% on skull X-ray

14 Retinoblastoma:

a) Is the most common intra-ocular malignancy in childhood
b) Ultrasound demonstrates a hypoechoic mass in the posterior globe
c) CT shows calcification in 90%
d) Is associated with pineoblastoma
e) Is bilateral in 66%

15 Causes of perinatal hydrocephalus include:

a) Aqueduct stenosis
b) Toxoplasmosis
c) Intraventricluar haemorrhage
d) Vein of Galen aneurysm
e) Choroid plexus papilloma

16 Regarding spinal anomalies:

a) The conus medullaris should reach the adult position by 12 weeks of age
b) Tethered cord is usually an isolated spinal anomaly
c) A filum measuring 3mm is within normal limits
d) Neurofibromatosis is the commonest cause of developmental scoliosis
e) Myelomeningocoele is usually associated with a Chiari I malformation

17 Regarding pancreatic development:

a) The tail, body and neck of the pancreas develop in the dorsal mesogastrium
b) The ventral pancreatic bud forms the uncinate process
c) The accessory pancreatic duct drains into the duodenum distal to the Ampulla of Vater
d) Annular pancreas is associated with Turner's syndrome
e) Pancreas divisum predisposes to chronic pancreatitis

18 In imaging of intussusception:

a) Plain radiographs can exclude the diagnosis
b) Small bowel (ileo-ileal) intussusception is usually due to a malignant cause
c) A target sign is seen on ultrasound
d) Ultrasound is highly sensitive and specific in the paediatric population
e) Air enema reduction should not exceed 120mmHg

19 Regarding abdominal cystic lesions in the newborn:

a) Enteric duplication cysts typically communicate with the bowel lumen
b) Duplication cysts are a known cause of gastrointestinal haemorrhage
c) Meconium pseudocyst is usually calcified
d) Choledochal cysts are associated with biliary atresia
e) Fluid-debris levels are typical of haemorrhage into an ovarian cyst

20 In imaging suspected acute appendicitis:

a) The appendix is retrocaecal in one third of cases
b) On ultrasound, luminal diameter of 8mm is normal
c) An inflamed appendix, if visualised, is usually non-compressible
d) Pseuodcyst peritoneii is a complication of appendiceal obstruction
e) A normal ultrasound excludes appendicitis as a diagnosis

21 Gallstones in the paediatric population may be secondary to:

a) Sickle cell disease
b) Cystic fibrosis
c) Crohn's disease
d) Ileal resection
e) Total parenteral nutrition

22 Concerning congenital diaphragmatic hernias:

a) Most congenital hernias are of the Morgagni type
b) Bochdalek hernias are usually left-sided
c) Defective closure of the pleuroperitoneal membranes leads to a Bochdalek hernia
d) Right-sided hernias may have a delayed presentation
e) Congenital cystic adenomatoid malformation is a differential diagnosis

23 Congenital bronchial atresia:

a) Bronchial development occurs during the 1st trimester
b) Bronchial atresia leads to distal air trapping
c) The right upper lobe is most commonly affected
d) Other congenital anomalies are frequently associated
e) A bronchocoele tends to radiate out from the hilar region

24 Regarding congenital lobar emphysema:

a) It commonly affects the lower lobes
b) Bilateral involvement is rare
c) Underlying vascular markings are present
d) The affected lobe is opaque after birth
e) It typically presents in the perinatal period

25 Regarding normal lung anatomy:

a) The azygous fissure contains 2 layers of pleura
b) The inferior accessory fissure separates the medial and anterior basal segments of a lower lobe
c) The right pulmonary artery passes posterior to the right main bronchus
d) The left superior pulmonary vein lies directly anterior to the left pulmonary artery
e) The anterior junctional line extends above the clavicles

26 In bronchopulmonary sequestration:

a) Intralobar sequestration typically presents in the neonatal period
b) Sequestered segments have delayed contrast enhancement on dynamic CT scanning
c) The condition may be diagnosed antenatally
d) Intralobar sequestered segments are covered by visceral pleura
e) There is usually communication with the bronchial tree

27 Concerning mediastinal masses in childhood:

a) Lymphomatous hilar lymph node enlargement usually occurs without mediastinal involvement
b) Paracardiac lymph nodes are a common site for primary haematological malignancy
c) Bronchogenic cysts are usually solitary
d) Pericardial cysts usually arise from the right cardiophrenic angle
e) Malignant teratomas are more common than benign teratomas

28 The following are features of cystic fibrosis:

a) Meconium ileus is the most common mode of presentation
b) Lung involvement predominates in the lower zones
c) Skull X-ray shows generalised hypoplasia of the paranasal sinuses
d) There is a known association with situs inversus
e) Contrast enemas are often therapeutic with meconium ileus

29 Regarding lung disease in premature neonates:

a) Respiratory distress syndrome is due to delayed clearance of lung fluid
b) Chest X-ray demonstrates hyperinflation of the lungs
c) Bilateral extensive consolidation is a feature
d) Mechanical ventilation is associated with pulmonary interstitial emphysema
e) Pulmonary interstitial emphysema may be unilateral

30 Causes of symmetrical periosteal reaction in childhood include:
- a) Leukaemia
- b) Juvenile idiopathic arthritis
- c) Caffey's disease
- d) Rickets
- e) Scurvy

31 Regarding hypoplastic left heart syndrome:
- a) Prenatal diagnosis is possible
- b) Pulmonary oligaemia is a feature
- c) The cardiac silhouette is small
- d) An ASD is commonly present
- e) Aortic coarctation is associated

32 Concerning the paediatric parotid gland:
- a) The parotid gland is hyperechoic to muscle on ultrasound
- b) Branchial cysts most often develop from the second branchial pouch
- c) Parotid haemangiomas are usually hypoehoic on ultrasound
- d) Warthin's tumours are bilateral in 25-50%
- e) Warthin's tumours are poorly defined masses

33 Radiological features of Wilms' tumours include:
- a) At CT, the tumour enhances to a greater degree than the surrounding renal parenchyma
- b) The tumour is hyperintense on T2 weighted MRI
- c) The tumour displaces midline structures
- d) Calcification is seen in up to 15% at CT
- e) Calcification, when present, tends to be curvilinear

34 Regarding ischaemic stroke in children:
- a) Intraparenchymal haemorrhage is usually spontaneous
- b) Cerebral MR changes are common in sickle cell disease
- c) Arterial dissection is rare
- d) *Varicella zoster* infection predisposes to basal ganglia infarcts
- e) Intracranial aneurysms are rare

35 Regarding congenital anomalies of the oesophagus:

a) The oesophagus and trachea are a single tube during early foetal life
b) Oesophageal atresia with a distal fistula is the most common form of atresia
c) Atelectasis and right upper lobe pneumonia are seen in 50% of oesophageal atresia
d) Oesophageal duplication is more common than ileal duplication
e) Aberrant right subclavian artery causes an anterior oesophageal impression on barium swallow examination

36 In duodenal atresia:

a) The double bubble sign may be seen on ultrasound examination
b) The double bubble sign is specific for duodenal atresia
c) Polyhydramnios is typical in the 3rd trimester
d) Over 50% are associated with Down's syndrome
e) Bowel gas is not seen distal to the atretic segment

37 Causes of dense metaphyseal bands include:

a) Normal variant
b) Treated leukaemia
c) Healing rickets
d) Lead toxicity
e) Hypervitaminosis D

38 Regarding congenital cardiac anomalies:

a) A left-sided SVC drains into the left atrium
b) A patent ductus arteriosus arises proximal to the left subclavian artery
c) In pulmonary artery sling, the aberrant left pulmonary artery passes between the trachea and oesophagus
d) An aortopulmonary window connects the descending thoracic aorta to the pulmonary trunk
e) Ebstein anomaly affects the tricuspid valve

39 Jaundice in childhood:

a) Physiological jaundice occurs in 60% of term infants
b) Gallbladder length may normally exceed that of the adjacent kidney
c) The normal paediatric pancreas is iso to hyperechoic compared to the liver
d) With biliary atresia, the intrahepatic bile ducts are dilated
e) On hepatobiliary scintigraphy, some small bowel activity may be seen in mild cases of biliary atresia

40 Causes of pulmonary plethora in the newborn include:

a) Transposition of the great arteries
b) Total anomalous pulmonary venous return
c) Tetralogy of Fallot
d) Pulmonary atresia
e) Patent ductus arteriosus

41 Medulloblastoma:

a) Is the most common paediatric CNS malignancy
b) Typically has a brief history (<3 months)
c) Typically arises within the cerebellar hemispheres
d) Is usually hypodense on pre-contrast CT
e) Post-contrast shows heterogenous enhancement

42 Regarding Sturge-Weber syndrome:

a) It involves a port-wine stain affecting the trigeminal nerve distribution
b) It is accompanied by leptomeningeal angiomas on the contralateral side
c) Underlying cortical calcification is common
d) Angiomas are more common over the frontotemporal regions
e) Cortical gliosis is a feature

43 Regarding calvarial masses in childhood:

a) The skull is the most common bone involved in Langerhans' cell histiocytosis
b) Sclerosis does not occur in Langerhans' cell histiocytosis
c) Monostotic fibrous dysplasia does not affect the skull
d) Neuroblastoma metastases rarely spread to the skull vault
e) Osteomas frequently arise from both the inner and outer calvarium

44 The radiological features of hepatocellular carcinoma include:

a) Calcification in up to 50% of cases
b) Portal vein involvement suggests an alternative diagnosis
c) Bone marrow metastases tend to be expansile
d) The tumour enhances during the arterial phase on dynamic CT
e) Signal drop out is typical with 'in and out of phase' MRI

45 Concerning anatomy and pathology of the orbit:

a) The optic foramen is formed by the greater wing of the sphenoid bone
b) The orbital margin is formed by the zygomatic, frontal and maxillary bones
c) Orbital pseudotumour frequently causes bone erosion
d) Orbital lymphoma typically affects the lacrimal gland
e) The lacrimal gland occupies a superolateral position within the orbital cavity

46 Features of dysostosis multiplex include:

a) Calvarial thickening
b) J shaped sella
c) Narrow anterior rib ends
d) Odontoid hypoplasia
e) Dysplastic femoral heads

47 Radiological features of Turner's syndrome (XO) include:

a) Tall stature
b) Shortened 5th metacarpal
c) Madelung's deformity
d) Enlarged medial femoral condyle
e) Osteoporosis

48 Regarding choledochal cysts:

a) They usually involve the cystic duct and gallbladder
b) There is normal orientation of the distal CBD and pancreatic duct
c) There is an association with gallbladder anomalies
d) The cyst does not communicate with common and intrahepatic ducts
e) There is increased incidence of cholangiocarcinoma

49 Regarding thyroglossal duct cysts:

a) The thyroglossal tract passes posterior to the hyoid bone
b) They are most commonly midline masses
c) Most are suprahyoid in location
d) Cysts are hypointense on T1 weighted MRI
e) Uncomplicated (non-inflamed) cysts do not enhance

50 Regarding brain development:

a) Adult sulcal pattern is obtained by 38 weeks gestation
b) On T2 weighted MRI, white matter maturation is seen as a reduction in signal intensity
c) Thinning of the corpus callosum is pathological
d) Myelination progresses uniformly throughout the brain
e) On MRI, the basilar cisterns remain prominent during infancy

1
a) False
b) True - overall, diaphyseal fractures are more common
c) True
d) False - interhemispheric subdural haematoma is a recognised feature
e) False - commonly occurs secondary to trivial twisting injuries

Rao, Carty. Non-Accidental Injury: Review of the Radiology. *Clinical Radiology* 1999; 54: 11-24.

2
a) True
b) True
c) False - equal sex incidence, but symptoms predominate in males
d) True - 60% by 10 years of age
e) True - intestinal obstruction is the second commonest

Levy, Hobbs. Meckel's Diverticulum: Radiologic Features with Pathologic Correlation. *RadioGraphics* 2004; 24(2): 565-85.

3
a) True
b) False - highest incidence between 3 months and 4 years of age
c) False - plain films may be normal in up to 50%
d) False - in children, 95% are idiopathic, with no lead point
e) True - as are peritonitis and hypotension

Radiology Review Manual. 5th edition. Dahnert. Lippincott, Williams and Wilkins, 2003: 835-7.

4
a) True
b) True
c) True
d) False - non-invasive, with a good prognosis
e) False - tumours are hyperintense on T2 sequences, and may be obscured by adjacent high signal urine

McHugh, Boothroyd. The Role of Radiology in Childhood Rhabdomyosarcoma. *Clinical Radiology* 1999; 54: 2-10.

5 a) True
b) True
c) True
d) True
e) True

Diagnostic Radiology. A Textbook of Medical Imaging. 4th edition. Grainger and Allison. Churchill Livingstone, 2001: 1743-7.

6 a) False - large, distended bladder
b) True - with cryptorchidism, distended bladder and dilated ureters
c) True
d) False
e) True

Textbook of Radiology and Imaging. 7th edition. Sutton. Churchill Livingstone, 2002: 1061.

7 a) True
b) True
c) False
d) True
e) False - cortical nephrocalcinosis

Aids to Radiological Differential Diagnosis. 4th edition. Chapman and Nakielny. W.B. Saunders, 2003: 313-4.

8 a) True
b) True
c) True - a narrow foramen magnum may cause obstructive hydrocephalus
d) False - posterior vertebral scalloping
e) False - relative lengthening of the fibula

Diagnostic Radiology. A Textbook of Medical Imaging. 4th edition. Grainger and Allison. Churchill Livingstone, 2001: 1973-4.

9 a) False - typically 8-17 years of age
b) True
c) True
d) True
e) False - an early sign of Perthes' disease

Radiology Review Manual. 5th edition. Dahnert. Lippincott, Williams and Wilkins, 2003: 72-3.

10 a) False - short limbs
b) True
c) False - increased bone density
d) True
e) True

Diagnostic Radiology. A Textbook of Medical Imaging. 4th edition. Grainger and Allison. Churchill Livingstone, 2001: 1986.

11 a) True
b) False - medial at 5 years, lateral at 13 years
c) False - a normal variant in up to 15%
d) False - capitate and hamate ossify in the 1st year; scaphoid in the 6th year
e) True

Applied Radiological Anatomy. Butler, Mitchell & Ellis. Cambridge University Press, 1999: 331-51.

12 a) True
b) True
c) True
d) True - also in pyknodysostosis, kinky hair syndrome, cleidocranial dysostosis, hypophosphatasia
e) False

Aids to Radiological Differential Diagnosis. 4th edition. Chapman and Nakielny. W.B. Saunders, 2003: 486.

13 a) True - myoclonic seizures in 80-100%
b) False - ventricular surface of the caudate nucleus
c) False - T2 weighted and FLAIR sequences
d) False - giant cell astrocytoma
e) True

Radiology Review Manual. 5th edition. Dahnert. Lippincott, Williams and Wilkins, 2003: 324-6.

14 a) True
b) False - hyperechoic mass within the globe
c) True
d) True - the trilateral retinoblastoma
e) True

Textbook of Radiology and Imaging. 7th edition. Sutton. Churchill Livingstone, 2002: 1591.

15 a) True
b) True
c) True
d) True
e) True

Pediatric Neuroimaging. 4th edition. Barkovich. Lippincott Williams & Wilkins, 2005: 659-703.

16 a) True
b) False - often associated with intraspinal abnormalities
c) False - 2mm at the L5/S1 level is considered thickened
d) True
e) False - Chiari II malformation

Redla, Sikdar, Saiffudin. MRI of Scoliosis. *Clinical Radiology* 2001; 56(5): 360-71.

17 a) True
b) True
c) False - proximal to the Ampulla of Vater
d) False - Down's syndrome, oesophageal atresia, imperforate anus, malrotation
e) True

Last's Anatomy, Regional and Applied. 10th Edition. Sinnatamby. Churchill Livingstone, 1999: 262-4.

18 a) False
b) False - usually benign aetiology, e.g. polyp, lipoma, coeliac disease
c) True
d) True
e) True

Byrne, Goeghegan, *et al.* The Imaging of Intussusception. *Clinical Radiology* 2005; 60: 39-46.

19 a) False
b) True - 10-20% contain ectopic gastric mucosa
c) True
d) True
e) True

Khong, Cheung, *et al.* Ultrasonography of Intra-abdominal Cystic Lesions in the Newborn. *Clinical Radiology* 2003; 58: 449-54.

20 a) False - 15% of cases
b) False - >6mm is abnormal
c) True
d) True
e) False

Diagnostic Radiology. A Textbook of Medical Imaging. 4th edition. Grainger and Allison. Churchill Livingstone, 2001.

21 a) True
b) True
c) True
d) True
e) True

Radiology Review Manual. 5th edition. Dahnert. Lippincott, Williams and Wilkins, 2003: 693-5.

22 a) False - 85-90% are Bochdalek hernias
b) True
c) True
d) True
e) True

Diagnostic Radiology. A Textbook of Medical Imaging. 4th edition. Grainger and Allison. Churchill Livingstone, 2001: 345-6

23 a) True
b) True
c) False - left upper lobe in 64%
d) False - an incidental finding in 50%, and usually isolated
e) True

Ward, Morcos. Congenital Bronchial Atresia. *Clinical Radiology* 1999; 54: 144-8.

24 a) False - lower lobes in only 2%. Left upper lobe most commonly
b) True
c) True
d) True
e) False - in 25%, presentation is delayed

Diagnostic Radiology. A Textbook of Medical Imaging. 4th edition. Grainger and Allison. Churchill Livingstone, 2001: The Respiratory System.

25 a) False - 4 layers
b) True
c) False - anterior
d) False - the bronchial tree lies in between the two structures
e) False - posterior junctional line

Applied Radiological Anatomy. Butler, Mithcell & Ellis. Cambridge University Press, 1999: 121-40.

26 a) False - later presentation is typical, with 50% asymptomatic
b) False - early or normal enhancement
c) True
d) True
e) False - communication may occur following infection

Radiology Review Manual. 5th edition. Dahnert. Lippincott, Williams and Wilkins, 2003: 471-3.

27 a) False - rare without mediastinal involvement
b) False - an important site of lymph node recurrence
c) True
d) True
e) False - benign cystic teratomas are the commonest mediastinal germ cell tumour

Diagnostic Radiology. A Textbook of Medical Imaging. 4th edition. Grainger and Allison. Churchill Livingstone, 2001: 354-71.

28 a) False - only 10-15% of cases present this way
b) False - upper zone predominance
c) False - frontal sinus hypoplasia. The remainder are normal
d) False - situs inversus and bronchiectasis are part of the immotile cilia syndrome
e) True

Radiology Review Manual. 5th edition. Dahnert. Lippincott, Williams and Wilkins, 2003: 481-2.

29 a) False - respiratory distress syndrome is due to surfactant deficiency
b) False - underexpansion is typical
c) True
d) True
e) True

Agrons, *et al.* Lung Disease in Premature Neonates: Radiologic - Pathologic Correlation. *RadioGraphics* 2005 25(4): 1047-73.

30 a) True - due to cortical involvement by tumour cells
b) True - in 25%
c) True
d) True
e) True

Aids to Radiological Differential Diagnosis. 4th edition. Chapman and Nakielny. W.B. Saunders, 2003: 38-9.

31 a) True
b) False - pulmonary venous hypertension
c) False - enlarged cardiac silhouette, notably the right atrium
d) True
e) True

Bardo, *et al.* Hypoplastic Left Heart Syndrome. *RadioGraphics* 2001; 21: 705-17.

32 a) True
b) True
c) True
d) False - only 10% are bilateral
e) False - well circumscribed, homogenous masses

Lowe, *et al.* Imaging of the Pediatric Parotid Gland and Peri-parotid Region. *Radiographics* 2001; 21: 1211-27.

33 a) False - lesser degree to surrounding renal parenchyma
b) True - isointense to renal parenchyma on T1 sequences
c) True
d) True
e) True

Aquisto, *et al.* Anaplastic Wilms' Tumour: Radiologic - Pathologic Correlation. *RadioGraphics* 2004; 24: 1709-13.

34 a) False - 70% have an underlying cause
b) True
c) False - this is a leading cause of paediatric stroke
d) True
e) True

Mini-Symposium: Stroke in Children. *Pediatric Radiology* 2004; 34: 2-23.

35 a) True - failure of division leads to tracheo-oesophageal fistula
b) True
c) True
d) False - ileal duplications are more common
e) False - posterior impression

Berrocal, *et al.* Congenital Anomalies of the Upper Gastrointestinal Tract. *RadioGraphics* 1999; 19: 855-72.

36 a) True - plain film, ultrasound and contrast studies may show this sign
b) False - also seen in duodenal stenosis, annular pancreas, preduodenal portal vein
c) True
d) False - one third are associated with trisomy 21
e) False - this may occur with a bifid CBD insertion

Traubici. The Double Bubble Sign. *Radiology* 2001; 220: 463-4.

37 a) True
b) True
c) True
d) True
e) True

Raber. The Dense Metaphyseal Band Sign. *Radiology* 1999; 211: 773-4.

38 a) False - drains into the right atrium via the coronary sinus
b) False - distal to the right subclavian artery
c) True
d) False - ascending thoracic aorta to the pulmonary trunk
e) True

Goo, *et al.* CT of Congenital Heart Disease: Normal Anatomy and Typical Pathologic Correlation. *RadioGraphics* 2003; 23: 147-65.

39 a) True
b) False
c) True
d) False
e) False - bowel activity excludes biliary atresia

Gubernil, *et al.* US Approach to Jaundice in Infants and Children. *RadioGraphics* 2000; 20: 173-95.

40 a) True
b) True
c) False - pulmonary oligaemia
d) False
e) True

Radiology Review Manual. 5th edition. Dahnert. Lippincott, Williams and Wilkins, 2003: 577.

41 a) True
b) True
c) False - cerebellar vermis
d) False - 89% show some degree of hyperattenuation pre-contrast
e) True

Koeller, Rushing. Medulloblastoma: A Comprehensive Review With Radiologic - Pathologic Correlation. *Radiographics* 2003; 23: 1613-37.

42 a) True
b) False - ipsilateral side
c) True
d) False - parieto-occipital region
e) True

Textbook of Radiology and Imaging. 7th edition. Sutton. Churchill Livingstone, 2002: 1738.

43 a) True
b) False - sclerosis at the edge of lesions may be seen post-treatment
c) False - both poly and monostotic fibrous dysplasia may affect the skull
d) False - a common site of metastatic involvement
e) False - rarely arise from the inner table

Willatt, Quaghebeur. Calvarial Masses of Infants and Children. A Radiological Approach. *Clinical Radiology* 2004; 59: 474-86.

44 a) False - up to 12% calcify
b) False
c) True
d) True
e) False - fatty change occurs in only 10%, hence signal drop out unlikely (unlike hepatic adenoma)

Yu, *et al.* Imaging Features of Hepatocellular Carcinoma. *Clinical Radiology* 2004; 59: 145-56.

45 a) False - lesser wing of sphenoid
b) True
c) False
d) True
e) True

Aviv, Miszkiel. Orbital Imaging: Part 2. Intraorbital Pathology. *Clinical Radiology* 2005; 60: 288-307.

46 a) True
b) True
c) False - narrow posterior ribs, with wide anterior rib ends
d) True
e) True

Diagnostic Radiology. A Textbook of Medical Imaging. 4th edition. Grainger and Allison. Churchill Livingstone, 2001: 1978-9.

47 a) False - short stature
b) False - short 4th metacarpal
c) True
d) True
e) True

Diagnostic Radiology. A Textbook of Medical Imaging. 4th edition. Grainger and Allison. Churchill Livingstone, 2001: 1993.

48 a) False
b) False - abnormal orientation is frequent
c) True
d) False - the cyst is in continuity with common and intrahepatic ducts
e) True

Radiology Review Manual. 5th edition. Dahnert. Lippincott, Williams and Wilkins, 2003: 692-3.

49 a) False - anterior to the hyoid bone
b) True - 75% are midline
c) False - most are infrahyoid
d) True
e) True

Radiology Review Manual. 5th edition. Dahnert. Lippincott, Williams and Wilkins, 2003: 394.

50 a) False - the sulci are formed, but will continue to obtain increasing depth
b) True
c) False - thinning between posterior body and splenium is a normal variant
d) False - pathways undergoing use mature first (e.g. motor pathways)
e) True

Pediatric Neuroimaging. 4th edition. AJ Barkovich. Lippincott Williams & Wilkins, 2005: 292-5.

Chapter 6
Central Nervous System and Head & Neck

1 The following are causes of a 'hair-on-end' appearance of the skull vault:

a) Haemangioma
b) Thalassaemia major
c) Hereditary spherocytosis
d) Rickets
e) Sickle cell anaemia

2 Secondary metastases to the brain:

a) Are the commonest cause of brain tumour in adults
b) Are usually multiple
c) Are supratentorial in 75-90%
d) Are usually hypodense on non-contrast CT
e) Are almost always high signal on T2 weighted MRI

3 Arachnoid cyst:

a) Is also known as leptomeningeal cyst
b) Most commonly occurs in the middle cranial fossa
c) One third are found in the posterior fossa
d) Can cause erosion of the calvarium
e) Can calcify

4 Concerning the submandibular space:

a) Anteriorly there is free communication between the submandibular space and the sublingual space
b) The superficial lobe of the submandibular gland lies inferolateral to mylohyoid
c) Intraglandular ducts are seen as linear hypoechoic structures on ultrasound
d) As with the parotid gland, normal lymph nodes are found within the submandibular gland
e) Stenson's duct exits in the floor of the mouth at the base of the frenulum

5 Pyogenic brain abscesses:

a) Most commonly occur secondary to a generalised septicaemia
b) Typically occur at the corticomedullary junction
c) Are more common in the occipital lobes than the frontal lobes
d) The most common causative organism is *Staphylococcus Spp.*
e) On CT have a smooth regular wall with relative thinning of the lateral wall

6 The following cause wide cranial sutures in children:

a) Subdural haematoma
b) Hypophosphatasia
c) Lead intoxication
d) Lymphoma
e) Neuroblastoma

7 Regarding subarachnoid haemorrhage:

a) It occurs secondary to arteriovenous malformation in 10% of cases
b) It is associated with subdural haemorrhage in 20% of cases
c) 15-20% of patients will have multiple aneurysms
d) Cerebral vasospasm is maximal from 48 to 72 hours after the event
e) MRI is the best modality for detecting early subarachnoid haemorrhage

8 **The following are true concerning MRI:**

a) The magnet is cooled with liquid helium
b) The shim coil lies within the gradient coil
c) Surface coils improve signal-to-noise ratio
d) Gadolinium is contraindicated in pregnancy
e) Gadolinium is contraindicated in patients with haemolytic anaemia

9 **The following are usually hyperdense to normal brain on CT:**

a) Medulloblastoma
b) Metastases
c) Acoustic neuroma
d) Epidermoid
e) Meningioma

10 **Klippel-Feil syndrome is associated with the following:**

a) Sprengel's deformity
b) Syringomyelia
c) Cranial asymmetry
d) Low posterior hair line
e) Schmorl nodes

11 **Chemodectomas:**

a) Are derived from chemoreceptor cells
b) Are bilateral in 20% of cases
c) Normally arise from the adventitial layer of the common carotid artery
d) Normally cause splaying of the internal and external carotid arteries
e) Normally cause narrowing of the internal and external carotid arteries

12 Concerning trauma to the skull:

a) Temporal bone fractures are most commonly transverse
b) Longitudinal temporal bone fractures often cause a sensorineural hearing loss
c) Transverse temporal bone fractures cause facial palsy in 30-50% of cases
d) Skull fracture is seen in 90% of cases of extradural haematomas
e) Subdural haematomas commonly cause diffuse swelling of the underlying hemisphere

13 Concerning orbital mass lesions:

a) 60-80% of children with retinoblastoma have bilateral tumours
b) On MRI, retinoblastoma usually enhances following intravenous gadolinium
c) Rhabdomyosarcoma of the orbit presents with rapid onset proptosis and visual loss
d) Inflammatory orbital pseudotumour involves the muscle tendons
e) 50% of patients with optic nerve glioma have neurofibromatosis Type 1

14 The following cause basal ganglia calcification:

a) Pseudopseudohypoparathyroidism
b) Hyperparathyroidism
c) Carbon monoxide poisoning
d) Toxoplasmosis
e) Cockayne's syndrome

15 Regarding cerebral interventional procedures:

a) An 8-French catheter is normally used
b) The right brachial artery is usually catheterised
c) Most interventional procedures are better done under local anaesthetic with mild sedation
d) Guidewires may safely remain within a catheter for up to 5 minutes without withdrawal and flushing
e) Injection of 25ml of contrast by hand in about 1.5 seconds is safe in the internal carotid artery

16 **The following are true of MRI:**

a) The net magnetisation factor rotates at the Larmor frequency
b) The Larmor frequency is 42.6 MHz at a magnetic field strength of 1.5 Tesla
c) The repetition time controls the amount of T1 weighting
d) T1 weighted images have an echo time less than 80ms
e) T1 recovery is also called longitudinal relaxation

17 **Multiple wormian bones are seen in the following:**

a) Down's syndrome
b) Osteogenesis imperfecta
c) Hyperphosphatasia
d) Osteopetrosis
e) Pyknodysostosis

18 **Concerning pineal region masses:**

a) Pineoblastomas are categorised as part of the primitive neuroectodermal tumour group
b) Pineoblastomas usually show poor enhancement
c) Pineal germinomas are associated with Parinaud's syndrome
d) Germinomas are 10 times more common in males than females
e) Germinomas are hypodense on unenhanced CT

19 **A generalised increase in skull vault density is seen in the following:**

a) Fibrous dysplasia
b) Fluorosis
c) Phenytoin therapy
d) Craniometaphyseal dysplasia
e) Myelofibrosis

20 Concerning pituitary adenomas:

a) Hormonally active pituitary adenomas are usually microadenomas
b) The normal posterior pituitary is hyperintense to grey matter on T1 weighted images
c) Prolactinoma is the most commonly encountered pituitary adenoma
d) They are five times more common than craniopharyngiomas
e) Immediately after injection of gadolinium, pituitary adenomas remain hypointense to grey matter on T1 weighted imaging

21 Causes of thickening of the skull calvarium include:

a) Acromegaly
b) Sickle cell anaemia
c) Rickets
d) Phenytoin
e) Hyperparathyroidism

22 Regarding meningiomas:

a) 1-4% are 'malignant'
b) Approximately 50% are parasagittal
c) The majority enhance homogenously
d) 40-60% calcify
e) The dural 'tail' sign is specific for meningioma

23 Concerning haemangioblastoma:

a) It is the commonest primary posterior fossa tumour in adults
b) Most are associated with von Hippel-Lindau syndrome
c) Calcification occurs in 20-30% of cases
d) It usually presents as a well defined cystic mass
e) Flow void may be seen on MRI

24 The following are true concerning central nervous system (CNS) infections:

a) Fungal infections present as meningitis more commonly than granuloma or abscess
b) Histoplasmosis tends to occur in the immunosuppressed
c) Mucormycosis tends to occur in the immunosuppressed
d) Cryptococcosis is the commonest CNS fungal infection
e) CT of the brain in cryptococcus infection is usually normal

25 Regarding differentiation between epidermoids and dermoids of the brain:

a) Both are formed due to enclosure of ectodermal elements when the neural tube closes
b) Epidermoids are more common
c) Epidermoids more closely resemble cerebrospinal fluid on MRI
d) Epidermoids may become malignant
e) Fat-fluid level on imaging is highly suggestive of dermoids

26 Concerning epiloia (tuberous sclerosis):

a) The classic triad of adenoma sebaceum, seizures and mental retardation occurs in 50% of cases
b) Subependymal giant cell astrocytoma typically occurs posteriorly in the 3rd ventricle
c) Heterotopic grey matter islands in white matter occur in the majority of patients
d) Most patients die from complications of renal involvement
e) It is associated with lymphangioleiomyomatosis

27 The following are true of colloid cysts:

a) They usually arise from the lateral ventricles
b) They typically obstruct the foramen of Monro
c) They are hyperdense on unenhanced CT in 60-80% of cases
d) They are usually high signal on T1 weighted MRI
e) They are associated with the Brun phenomenon

28 Concerning parasitic CNS infections:

a) The brain is involved in 10-20% of cases of hydatid disease
b) Most patients with cysticercosis develop seizures
c) Hydatid disease of the brain mostly involves the posterior fossa
d) Toxoplasmosis is often confused with CNS lymphoma
e) Grape-like clustered lesions in the basal cisterns are seen in cysticercosis

29 Concerning cerebellopontine angle masses:

a) Meningiomas are the second commonest cerebellopontine angle mass
b) Meningiomas are typically brighter on T2 weighted MRI than T1
c) Meningiomas commonly cause expansion of the internal auditory canal
d) Epidermoids have the same signal as cerebrospinal fluid on MRI
e) Acoustic neuroma usually enhance poorly on post-contrast scans

30 A small pituitary fossa is caused by the following:

a) Radiotherapy as a child
b) Dystrophia myotonica
c) Nelson's syndrome
d) Hypopituitarism
e) Achondroplasia

31 Indications for MRI in stroke include:

a) Normal CT
b) Investigation of venous thrombosis
c) Investigation of arterial dissection
d) Supratentorial infarcts
e) Detection of reversible ischaemia

32 The following are true of the signal characteristics of intracerebral haematoma on MRI:

a) In the first 12 hours the haematoma is high signal on T1 weighted images
b) Intracellular methaemoglobin is high signal on T2 weighted images
c) Extracellular methaemoglobin is low signal on T2 weighted images
d) Haemosiderin is low signal on T1 weighted images
e) Deoxyhaemoglobin is low signal on T2 weighted images

33 Posterior scalloping of vertebral bodies is caused by the following:

a) Ependymoma
b) Acromegaly
c) Lipoma
d) Syringomyelia
e) Down's syndrome

34 Concerning brain herniation:

a) Uncal herniation is the commonest type
b) Uncal herniation normally causes a 'blown out' pupil
c) Subfalcine herniation causes enlargement of the adjacent lateral ventricle
d) Uncal herniation causes infarction of the posterior cerebral artery
e) Transtentorial herniation causes infarction of the posterior inferior cerebellar artery

35 Concerning otosclerosis:

a) It usually presents in infancy
b) It is more common in females
c) Stapedial otosclerosis causes a progressive sensorineural hearing loss
d) A lucent halo is seen around the cochlea on CT in the late phase of cochlear otosclerosis
e) Cochlear otosclerosis is more commonly seen than stapedial otosclerosis

36 Concerning orbital anatomy:

a) The inferior orbital fissure communicates with the pterygopalatine fossa and the masticator space
b) There are 7 extra-ocular muscles
c) All the extra-ocular muscles arise from a common fibrous ring, the annulus of Zinn
d) The ophthalmic artery lies inferior to the optic nerve in the optic foramen
e) The levator palpebrae superioris can easily be identified on MRI

37 Concerning the differences between cortical contusions and diffuse axonal injury (DAI):

a) Patients with cortical contusions are much less likely to have had loss of consciousness
b) Patients with cortical contusions usually have a better prognosis
c) Cortical contusions are more commonly haemorrhagic than DAI
d) CT is the best modality to diagnose acute DAI
e) Most patients with DAI suffer immediate loss of consciousness

38 Concerning non-accidental injury (NAI):

a) Skull fracture is the commonest NAI
b) Subdural haemorrhage is the commonest intracranial complication
c) Different ages of subdural haemorrhage seen on CT is pathognomonic of NAI
d) NAI-associated fracture usually affects the parietal bone
e) NAI accounts for half of deaths from head trauma in children less than 2 years of age

39 Concerning brain infarction:

a) Peak time for haemorrhagic transformation is 3-5 days post-infarct
b) Maximal brain swelling is seen on imaging on days 3-7 post-infarct
c) Gyral enhancement peaks from days 7-14 on CT
d) The hyperdense artery sign is usually seen within the first 2 hours post-infarct
e) The insular ribbon sign is usually seen within the first 2 hours post-infarct

40 Regarding Fong disease:
a) It is an autosomal recessive disorder
b) Hypoplasia of the fingernails of the thumb and index finger is a feature
c) Bilateral posterior iliac horns are diagnostic, but only seen in one third of patients
d) It may be associated with recurrent dislocation of the patella
e) It is associated with renal osteodystrophy

41 Concerning differences between primary CNS lymphoma and toxoplasmosis:
a) High signal on T2 weighted MRI favours lymphoma
b) Subependymal extension across the corpus callosum is more likely to occur in toxoplasmosis
c) Toxoplasmosis is more frequently multiple
d) The lesions are usually smaller in lymphoma
e) Ring enhancement following contrast administration favours lymphoma

42 Regarding contrast media:
a) Nephrotoxicity is predisposed in patients with multiple myeloma
b) Contrast potentiates blood clotting and platelet aggregation
c) Prophylactic haemodialysis lowers the risk of contrast media nephrotoxicity in patients with pre-existing renal impairment
d) Intravenous infusion of 0.9% saline lowers the risk of contrast media nephrotoxicity in patients with pre-existing renal impairment
e) Haemofiltration lowers the risk of contrast media nephrotoxicity in patients with pre-existing renal impairment

43 Regarding osmotic myelinolysis:
a) It is caused by rapid correction of hypernatraemia
b) It affects the pons most commonly
c) MRI typically shows abnormality within 24 hours
d) On MRI there is hyperintensity on T2 weighted imaging
e) There is a good response to treatment

44 The following structures pass through the jugular foramen:

a) Tenth cranial nerve
b) Twelfth cranial nerve
c) Internal jugular vein
d) Superior petrosal sinus
e) Ascending pharyngeal artery

45 Cerebellar medulloblastoma:

a) Is the commonest paediatric brain tumour
b) Is more common in females
c) 75% of patients are less than 15 years of age
d) Calcification occurs in 40-50%
e) Is associated with basal cell carcinomas

46 The following are causes of intra-orbital calcification:

a) Haemangioma
b) Neurofibroma
c) Rhabdomyosarcoma
d) Coat's disease
e) Adenocarcinoma of the lacrimal gland

47 Glucagon:

a) Has an immediate onset of action
b) Is less potent than buscopan
c) Has a duration of action of 30 minutes
d) Is contraindicated in pregnant or breastfeeding women
e) Decreases peristalsis in the oesophagus

48 Regarding acquired immune deficiency syndrome (AIDS) of the CNS:

a) 60-80% of patients with AIDS will develop neurologic symptoms
b) The cortical grey matter is usually spared in HIV encephalitis
c) AIDS dementia complex occurs in approximately 40-50% of patients with AIDS
d) Progressive multifocal leukoencephalopathy does not occur in patients with normal immunity
e) Primary CNS lymphoma is by far the commonest intracranial tumour in AIDS

49 The following are true concerning chemical shift artefact in MRI:

a) It occurs in the frequency encoding direction
b) It increases with decreasing field strength
c) Increasing the bandwidth decreases the risk of chemical shift artefact
d) A dark line is seen adjacent to fat
e) Is used in diagnosing certain fat-containing lesions

50 Concerning vascular masses of the head and neck:

a) High-flow vascular malformations are normally treated with percutaneous sclerotherapy
b) Infantile haemangiomas usually warrant intervention
c) Pre-operative embolisation of juvenile angiofibroma reduces blood loss at surgery but may predispose to recurrence
d) Extracranial external carotid artery aneurysms are most frequently secondary to atherosclerotic disease
e) Haemangiopericytomas are benign tumours that may be located in the soft tissues of the neck

1 a) True
b) True
c) True
d) False
e) True

Aids to Radiological Differential Diagnosis. 4th edition. Chapman and Nakielny. W.B. Saunders, 2003: 489.

2 a) False - approximately two thirds of brain tumours are primary tumours, whereas one third are secondary metastases
b) True
c) True - however, from renal cell carcinoma are usually located in the posterior fossa
d) True - however, haemorrhagic metastases may be hyperdense precontrast
e) False - variable signal intensity on T2 weighted images

Radiology Review Manual. 5th edition. Dahnert. Lippincott, Williams and Wilkins, 2003: 302-3.
Fundamentals of Diagnostic Radiology. 2nd edition. Brant and Helms. Lippincott, Williams and Wilkins, 1999: 126-8.

3 a) True - this is the acquired form, usually secondary to trauma or surgery
b) True - 50%
c) True
d) True - the inner table
e) False

Radiology Review Manual. 5th edition. Dahnert. Lippincott, Williams and Wilkins, 2003: 262.

4 a) False - posteriorly
b) True
c) False - linear hyperechoic structures
d) False - due to early glandular encapsulation normal lymph nodes are not found within the submandibular gland
e) False - Wharton's duct

Howlett, *et al.* Imaging of the Submandibular Space. *Clinical Radiology* 2004; 59: 1070-8.

5 a) False - 32% occur due to generalised septicaemia from for example, a lung abscess or pneumonia. However, 41% occur secondary to extension from paranasal sinus infection
b) True
c) False
d) False - anaerobic *Streptococcus Spp.*
e) False - relative thinning of medial wall due to poorer blood supply of white matter. This predisposes to rupture of the abscess medially into the ventricular system

Radiology Review Manual. 5th edition. Dahnert. Lippincott, Williams and Wilkins, 2003: 257.

6 a) True - only seen in children less than 10 years of age
b) True
c) True
d) True
e) True - also +/- sunray spiculation

Aids to Radiological Differential Diagnosis. 4th edition. Chapman and Nakielny. W.B. Saunders, 2003: 421.

7 a) True
b) False - 5%
c) True
d) False - 5-17 days
e) False - may not be seen on MRI for 48 hours. When haemorrhage occurs, oxyHb is converted to deoxyHb at a rate depending on oxygen tension and local pH. This can be delayed when oxygen-containing CSF surrounds the haemorrhage. This is why it is difficult to detect subarachnoid haemorrhage on MRI

Radiology Review Manual. 5th edition. Dahnert. Lippincott, Williams and Wilkins, 2003: 320-1.

8 a) True
b) False - outside it
c) True
d) True
e) True

Physics for Medical Imaging. Farr, Allisy-Roberts. Bailliere Tindell, 1996: 215-51.

9
a) True - in 80%
b) False - usually hypodense
c) False - usually isodense but enhances avidly
d) False - hypodense
e) True

Aids to Radiological Differential Diagnosis. 4th edition. Chapman and Nakielny. W.B. Saunders, 2003: 425.

10
a) True - in 25-40%
b) True
c) True
d) True
e) False

Radiology Review Manual. 5th edition. Dahnert. Lippincott, Williams and Wilkins, 2003: 212.

11
a) False - chemodectoma is a misnomer
b) False - 5%
c) True
d) True
e) False

Radiology Review Manual. 5th edition. Dahnert. Lippincott, Williams and Wilkins, 2003: 388.

12
a) False - 75% are longitudinal
b) False - conductive hearing loss
c) True - this is often complete
d) True
e) True - therefore causing more mass effect than would be expected

Fundamentals of Diagnostic Radiology. 2nd edition. Brant and Helms. Lippincott, Williams and Wilkins, 1999: 49-66.

13 a) False - 20-40%, and this is most often the autosomal dominant type
b) True
c) False - vision is preserved
d) True
e) False - 25%. 15% of patients with neurofibromatosis Type 1 have optic nerve glioma

Aids to Radiological Differential Diagnosis. 4th edition. Chapman and Nakielny. W.B. Saunders, 2003: 375-83.

14 a) True
b) True
c) True
d) True
e) True - autosomal recessive demyelinating disease associated with deafness and dwarfism

Aids to Radiological Differential Diagnosis. 4th edition. Chapman and Nakielny. W.B. Saunders, 2003: 430.

15 a) False - 5 or 6-French
b) False - right femoral artery
c) False - general anaesthetic is best for cerebral interventional procedures
d) False - up to 1 minute
e) False - 7ml

A Guide to Radiological Procedures. 4th edition. Chapman and Nakielny. W.B. Saunders, 2001: 302-5.

16 a) True
b) False - 63.9 MHz
c) True
d) False - less than 20ms
e) True

Physics for Medical Imaging. Farr, Allisy-Roberts. Bailliere Tindell, 1996: 215-51.

17 a) True
b) True
c) False - hypophosphatasia
d) False
e) True

Aids to Radiological Differential Diagnosis. 4th edition. Chapman and Nakielny. W.B. Saunders, 2003: 486.

18 a) True - they are similar to medulloblastomas
b) False - avidly enhance
c) True - paralysis of upward gaze
d) True
e) False - isodense or hyperdense

Fundamentals of Diagnostic Radiology. 2nd edition. Brant and Helms. Lippincott, Williams and Wilkins, 1999: 128-30.

19 a) True
b) True - calcification of muscle attachments is also seen
c) True
d) True - associated with metaphyseal splaying of the long bones
e) True - the spleen is greatly enlarged

Aids to Radiological Differential Diagnosis. 4th edition. Chapman and Nakielny. W.B. Saunders, 2003: 482.

20 a) True - 75% of pituitary adenomas are hormonally active
b) True
c) True
d) True
e) True - they become isointense or hyperintense after half an hour

Fundamentals of Diagnostic Radiology. 2nd edition. Brant and Helms. Lippincott, Williams and Wilkins, 1999: 130-2.

21 a) True - also causes an enlarged sella
b) True - due to extramedullary haematopoesis
c) False - causes thinning of skull
d) True
e) False - causes thinning of skull

Aids to Radiological Differential Diagnosis. 4th edition. Chapman and Nakielny. W.B. Saunders, 2003: 484-5.

22 a) True - i.e. invade local brain parenchyma
b) True
c) True - 10% have low attenuation areas representing necrosis
d) False - 20%
e) False - seen in 60% of meningiomas but it is not specific

Fundamentals of Diagnostic Radiology. 2nd edition. Brant and Helms. Lippincott, Williams and Wilkins, 1999: 133-7.

23 a) True
b) False - 4-20% are associated with von Hippel-Lindau syndrome
c) False - calcification is very rare
d) True - in 40% presents as solid mass
e) True - from the vascular pedicle of the mural nodule associated with cystic haemangioblastoma

Fundamentals of Diagnostic Radiology. 2nd edition. Brant and Helms. Lippincott, Williams and Wilkins, 1999: 137.

24 a) True
b) False - endemic
c) True
d) True
e) True - reflecting mild meningeal involvement

Fundamentals of Diagnostic Radiology. 2nd edition. Brant and Helms. Lippincott, Williams and Wilkins, 1999: 143-67.

25 a) True
b) True
c) True
d) False - both are benign and slow growing
e) True

Fundamentals of Diagnostic Radiology. 2nd edition. Brant and Helms. Lippincott, Williams and Wilkins, 1999: 137-8.

26 a) False - 30%
b) False - it occurs anteriorly in the region of the foramen of Monro
c) True - 93%
d) True - 75% of patients die from complications of renal failure by 20 years of age
e) True - in 1% of cases

Radiology Review Manual. 5th edition. Dahnert. Lippincott, Williams and Wilkins, 2003: 325-6.

27 a) False - typically 3rd ventricle
b) True
c) False - 50% hyperdense. 50% isodense
d) True
e) True - acute severe headache reproduced by patient tilting head forward. In this position the cyst may obstruct the foramen of Monro

Fundamentals of Diagnostic Radiology. 2nd edition. Brant and Helms. Lippincott, Williams and Wilkins, 1999: 139.

28 a) False - 1-4%
b) True - 90%
c) False - usually supratentorial CSF-density lesions in middle cerebral artery territory
d) True
e) True

Fundamentals of Diagnostic Radiology. 2nd edition. Brant and Helms. Lippincott, Williams and Wilkins, 1999: 150-2.

29 a) True
b) False - less bright on T2 weighted MRI
c) False - usually no expansion
d) True
e) False - enhances avidly

Aids to Radiological Differential Diagnosis. 4th edition. Chapman and Nakielny. W.B. Saunders, 2003: 469.

30 a) True
b) True - hereditary condition of early adult life characterised by frontal baldness, cataracts, testicular atrophy and thickening of the skull with large frontal sinuses
c) False - this is seen post-adrenalectomy for Cushing's syndrome and causes an expanded pituitary fossa
d) True
e) False - this causes a J-shaped sella

Aids to Radiological Differential Diagnosis. 4th edition. Chapman and Nakielny. W.B. Saunders, 2003: 458-9.

31 a) True - MRI is more sensitive than CT for the diagnosis of early ishaemic stroke and small vascular insults
b) True - loss of the normal flow void within a dural sinus or cerebral vein may indicate thrombosis
c) True
d) False - however, MRI is vastly superior to CT in evaluation of the posterior fossa
e) True

Aids to Radiological Differential Diagnosis. 4th edition. Chapman and Nakielny. W.B. Saunders, 2003: 401.

32 a) False - intermediate signal intensity. At this stage it is bright on T2 weighted images due to oxyhaemoglobin
b) False - low signal
c) False - high signal
d) True
e) True

Aids to Radiological Differential Diagnosis. 4th edition. Chapman and Nakielny. W.B. Saunders, 2003: 404.

33 a) True - especially of the filum terminale and conus
b) True
c) True
d) True - especially if the onset is before 30 years of age
e) False - but causes anterior scalloping of vertebral bodies

Aids to Radiological Differential Diagnosis. 4th edition. Chapman and Nakielny. W.B. Saunders, 2003: 87-8.

34 a) False - subfalcine herniation is the most common
b) True - due to compression of 3rd cranial nerve
c) False - compression of the adjacent lateral ventricle and enlargement of the contralateral one due to obstruction at the level of the foramen of Monro
d) True
e) True

Fundamentals of Diagnostic Radiology. 2nd edition. Brant and Helms. Lippincott, Williams and Wilkins, 1999: 61-3.

35 a) False - adolescents and young adults
b) True
c) False - progressive conductive hearing loss
d) False - this is seen in the early phase. Later bony proliferation and sclerosis occur
e) False - cochlear otosclerosis 10-20%. Stapedial otosclerosis 80-90%

Radiology Review Manual. 5th edition. Dahnert. Lippincott, Williams and Wilkins, 2003: 387.

36 a) True
b) True - four rectus muscles comprise the muscle cone, the levator palpebrae superioris and the inferior and superior oblique muscles
c) False - all except inferior oblique muscle
d) True
e) False - with the superior rectus muscle is often referred to as the superior muscle complex

Aviv, Casselman. Orbital Imaging: Part 1. Normal Anatomy. *Clinical Radiology* 2005; 60: 271-87.

37 a) True
b) True
c) True
d) False - much better seen on MRI than CT
e) True

Fundamentals of Diagnostic Radiology. 2nd edition. Brant and Helms. Lippincott, Williams and Wilkins, 1999: 56-60.

38 a) False - second commonest after long bone fracture
b) True
c) False - they do have a propensity to rebleed if spontaneous
d) False - usually occipital
e) False - 80%

Fundamentals of Diagnostic Radiology. 2nd edition. Brant and Helms. Lippincott, Williams and Wilkins, 1999: 66-7.

39 a) False - 1-2 weeks post-infarct
b) True
c) True
d) False - at 2-6 hours
e) False - at 2-6 hours

Fundamentals of Diagnostic Radiology. 2nd edition. Brant and Helms. Lippincott, Williams and Wilkins, 1999: 79-100.

40 a) False - rare autosomal dominant disorder characterised by symmetrical meso- and ectodermal anomalies
b) True - also spooning, splitting and ridging of fingernails
c) False - diagnostic but seen in 80% of patients
d) True - a feature is fragmentation, hypoplasia or absence of the patella
e) True

Radiology Review Manual. 5th edition. Dahnert. Lippincott, Williams and Wilkins, 2003: 124-5.

41 a) False - toxoplasmosis
b) False
c) True
d) False
e) False - toxoplasmosis

Fundamentals of Diagnostic Radiology. 2nd edition. Brant and Helms. Lippincott, Williams and Wilkins, 1999: 164-6.

42 a) True
b) False - it impairs it
c) False
d) True - (1ml/kg body weight/hr) starting 4 hours before contrast injection and continuing for at least 12 hours afterwards
e) True

A Guide to Radiological Procedures. 4th edition. Chapman and Nakielny. W.B. Saunders 2001: 30-40.
Morcos. Prevention of Contrast Media Nephrotoxicity. *Clinical Radiology* 2004; 59: 381-9.

43 a) False - caused by rapid correction or overcorrection of severe hyponatraemia. Usually occurs in a comatose patient following prolonged intravenous fluid administration. 60-70% occurs in chronic alcoholics
b) True
c) False - MRI becomes positive 1-2 weeks post-onset of symptoms
d) True
e) False - 5-10% survival rate beyond 6 months

Radiology Review Manual. 5th edition. Dahnert. Lippincott, Williams and Wilkins, 2003: 266.

44 a) True
b) False - passes through its own canal, the hypoglossal canal
c) True
d) False - inferior petrosal sinus, which drains to the internal jugular vein
e) True

Anatomy for Diagnostic Imaging. 2nd Edition. Ryan, McNichols and Eustace. W.B Saunders, 2004: 7.

45 a) False - second commonest paediatric tumour. Is second only to astrocytoma. However, it is the commonest paediatric posterior fossa tumour

b) False - more common in males

c) True - peak occurrences are from 4-8 years and 15-35 years of age

d) False - calcification occurs in up to 20% of patients. Cystic change or necrosis occurs in up to 50%. Medulloblastomas are usually solid hyperdense masses on CT. On MRI they are usually hypointense to grey matter on T1 weighting and have an extremely variable appearance on T2 weighting. Oedema is almost always seen

e) True - high incidence of medulloblastoma is seen in children with Gorlin's syndrome (basal cell naevus syndrome)

Fundamentals of Diagnostic Radiology. 2nd edition. Brant and Helms. Lippincott, Williams and Wilkins, 1999: 122.
Radiology Review Manual. 5th edition. Dahnert. Lippincott, Williams and Wilkins, 2003: 50.

46 a) True - only rarely have calcified phleboliths

b) True - rarely

c) False

d) False - but indistinguishable from non-calcified retinoblastoma

e) True - may calcify

Aids to Radiological Differential Diagnosis. 4th edition. Chapman and Nakielny. W.B. Saunders, 2003: 386.

47 a) False - onset is in one minute

b) False - more potent

c) False - 15 minutes

d) False - safe

e) False - however, buscopan does and is therefore preferred when assessing for oesophageal varices

A Guide to Radiological Procedures. 4th edition. Chapman and Nakielny. W.B. Saunders, 2001: 54-99.

48 a) False - 40%
b) True
c) False - 7-15%
d) True
e) True

Fundamentals of Diagnostic Radiology. 2nd edition. Brant and Helms. Lippincott, Williams and Wilkins, 1999: 162-7.

49 a) True
b) False - decreases
c) True - but this will decrease signal-to-noise ratio
d) True
e) True

Physics for Medical Imaging. Farr, Allisy-Roberts. Bailliere Tindell, 1996: 215-51.

50 a) False - intra-arterial embolisation with possible surgical excision
b) False - they spontaneously involute. Although non-involuting cases are described in 5% of cases
c) True
d) False - most frequently secondary to trauma. But may also result from infection, congenital vascular anomalies and atherosclerotic disease
e) False - may be malignant

Connor, Langdon. Vascular Masses of the Head and Neck. *Clinical Radiology* 2005; 60: 856-68.

Section II

Practice Papers

In the exam a negative marking system is used whereby +1 mark is given for every question answered correctly, -1 mark for every question answered incorrectly and 0 marks for every question answered as a 'don't know'.

The duration of each question paper and the number of MCQs in each is shown below:

Module 1: Cardiothoracic and Vascular	40 questions	2 hours
Module 2: Musculoskeletal and Trauma	30 questions	1.5 hours
Module 3: Gastrointestinal	40 questions	2 hours
Module 4: Genitourinary, Adrenal, Obstetrics & Gynaecology and Breast	30 questions	1.5 hours
Module 5: Paediatrics	30 questions	1.5 hours
Module 6: Central Nervous System and Head & Neck	30 questions	1.5 hours

Paper 1

Cardiothoracic and Vascular

1 The following surgical procedures are used in the treatment of the associated conditions:

a) Aorticopulmonary window repair - tetralogy of Fallot
b) Blalock-Taussig shunt - transposition of the great vessels
c) Fontan procedure - tricuspid atresia
d) Mustard procedure - transposition of great vessels
e) Norwood procedure - hypoplastic left heart syndrome

2 The following decrease signal-to-noise ratio in MRI:

a) 3D imaging
b) Thinner slices
c) Using T2 rather than T1 weighted images
d) Using a shorter echo time
e) Using spin-echo rather than gradient-echo sequences

3 Plain radiograph findings of a patient with Eisenmenger's syndrome include:

a) Constriction of the pulmonary trunk
b) Dilatation of the peripheral pulmonary arteries
c) Enlargement of the right ventricle
d) Dilatation of the pulmonary veins
e) Left ventricle returning to normal size

4 Regarding pulmonary arterial embolisation:

a) The principal indication is for the occlusion of pulmonary arteriovenous malformations
b) Pulmonary embolisation is performed with particulate emboli
c) Pulmonary arteriovenous malformations must be occluded as close to the neck as possible
d) Pulmonary arteriovenous malformations seen on chest X-ray as opacities remain unchanged in size despite successful embolisation
e) 80-90% of pulmonary arteriovenous malformations are associated with hereditary haemorrhagic telangiectasia

5 Regarding single photon emission tomography for myocardial perfusion studies:

a) Technetium-99m is the most commonly used radionuclide
b) Infarction can be differentiated from ischaemia
c) Stress and resting images are obtained
d) Imaging begins 30 minutes after injection of radionuclide
e) The half life of technetium-99m is 30 minutes

6 An aberrant left pulmonary artery:

a) Passes below the right main bronchus
b) Passes posterior to the oesophagus on its way to the left lung
c) Is associated with a patent ductus arteriosus
d) Causes deviation of the trachea to the right
e) Is associated with an elevated left hilum

7 Regarding Takayasu's arteritis:

a) The mean interval between symptom onset and diagnosis is 2-4 months
b) External carotid artery branches are most commonly affected
c) It is a recognised cause of fusiform aortic aneurysms
d) Stenotic lesions are more commonly seen in the thoracic than abdominal aorta
e) Ultrasound of the proximal common carotid artery shows circumferential thickening of the vessel wall

8 Regarding pericardial disease:

a) A pericardium of 3mm thickness is normal
b) Rheumatoid arthritis is a cause of pericarditis
c) Elevation of the jugular venous pressure on inspiration is a sign of chronic pericarditis
d) In chronic pericarditis, CT shows curvature of the interventricular septum to the right
e) Renal failure is a cause of pericardial effusion

9 Features of cardiac myxoma include:

a) Commonest location is the right atrium
b) Association with Carney complex
c) Reduced signal on T2 weighted spin-echo MRI images
d) Commonest site of metastases is the liver
e) The majority show homogenous contrast enhancement on CT

10 The following are signs of an aortic graft infection:

a) Perigraft haematoma seen at 2-3 weeks post-surgery
b) Ectopic gas seen at 5-6 weeks post-surgery
c) >5mm soft tissue between graft and surrounding wrap after 7 weeks postoperative
d) Focal bowel wall thickening adjacent to graft
e) Focal discontinuity of calcified aneurysmal wrap

11 Regarding polysplenia syndrome:

a) It is more commonly associated with congenital heart disease than asplenia syndrome
b) Dextrocardia is seen in 30-40%
c) A large azygous vein which mimics the aortic arch is a specific feature
d) Bilateral minor fissures are seen
e) Bilateral superior vena cavas are seen in 40-50%

12 Regarding metastases to the heart and pericardium:

a) Primary cardiac tumours are more common than metastases to the heart and pericardium
b) Lymphoma is the commonest primary tumour to metastasise to the heart
c) Melanoma metastases spread via the lymphatics
d) Melanoma metastases appear as low signal intensity lesions on T1 weighted MRI images
e) More than 50% of cases of mesothelioma invade the pericardium

13 Regarding popliteal artery disease:

a) The popliteal artery is located between the two heads of the gastrocnemius muscle
b) The popliteal artery is considered aneurysmal if its diameter exceeds 7mm
c) Popliteal artery aneurysms are bilateral in 10-15%
d) In popliteal artery entrapment syndrome, patients are usually elderly females
e) Primary treatment for popliteal artery entrapment syndrome is vascular stenting

14 Features of polyarteritis nodosa include:

a) Necrotising vasculitis involving the small and medium-sized arteries
b) Involvement of kidneys in 70-80%
c) Multiple aneurysms
d) Luminal irregularities
e) Involvement of small veins

15 Regarding positron emission tomography (PET):

a) 18F fluorodeoxyglucose is the radioisotope most commonly used
b) Two times more events are detected with PET per decay than single photon imaging
c) Image noise is decreased by increasing the scan time
d) Benign and malignant pleural effusions can be differentiated on PET
e) Tuberculosis is a recognised cause of a false positive

16 The following statements about endovascular repair of thoracic/abdominal aortic aneuryms are true:

a) The commonest complication after stent graft implantation is graft thrombosis
b) Type 2 endoleak arises due to defects of the graft
c) Type 3 endoleak is the commonest type
d) Shower embolism occurs less frequently after endovascular than open aneurysm repair
e) Aortic dissection is a complication arising due to retrograde injury from introduction of stent delivery systems

17 Thymoma:

a) Is associated with myasthenia gravis
b) Is associated with hypogammaglobulinaemia
c) Commonly presents with SVC obstruction
d) Commonly presents in children
e) Is isointense to skeletal muscle on T1 weighted MRI images

18 Causes of cardiac calcification include:

a) Endocardial fibroelastosis
b) Endomyocardial fibrosis
c) Chronic renal failure
d) Mediastinal radiotherapy
e) Left ventricular aneurysm

19 Regarding superior mesenteric angiography:

a) Cobra catheters have 1 end hole and 4-6 side holes
b) Gastrointestinal ischaemia is an indication
c) When carried out for gastrointestinal bleeding, blood loss of 0.5ml per minute can be identified if the patient is bleeding at the time
d) Examination is perfomed with the patient in a prone position
e) When examined with the inferior mesenteric artery, the superior mesenteric artery should be examined first

20 Regarding cardiomyopathies:

a) Alcoholism is a recognised cause of restrictive cardiomyopathy
b) Amyloidosis is a recognised cause of dilated cardiomyopathy
c) Hypertrophic cardiomyopathy is inherited in an autosomal recessive manner
d) Mitral stenosis is a feature of hypertrophic cardiomyopathy
e) In dilated cardiomyopathy the left ventricle is usually spared

21 Regarding thoracic anatomy:

a) The superior accessory fissure separates the apical segment of the right lower lobe from the other segments
b) The left transverse fissure is seen in 15-20% of post mortem specimens
c) The right major fissure is more vertically orientated than the left
d) The minor fissure is absent in 25-30%
e) The minor fissure meets the right major fissure at the level of the 6th rib in the mid-clavicular line

22 Loss of clarity of the right heart border silhouette can be due to:

a) Pneumothorax on a supine radiograph
b) Pectus excavatum
c) Middle lobe collapse
d) Right lower lobe collapse
e) Asbestosis

23 The following are anterior relations of the trachea:

a) Inferior thyroid veins
b) Left recurrent laryngeal nerve
c) Left brachiocephalic vein
d) Sternohyoid muscle
e) Arch of the azygous vein

24 Regarding endovascular management of disorders of the thoracic aorta:

a) Zenith endograft is a self-expanding stent graft suitable for treating thoracic aortic aneurysms
b) Imaging criteria for stent grafting are upper and lower zones of relatively normal calibre aorta of at least 5mm
c) Brachial artery access is used
d) Endovascular treatment is suitable for ascending but not descending thoracic aortic aneurysms
e) The diameter of the stent device should be oversized by 10-20% of the diameter of normal aorta

25 Regarding extralobular bronchopulmonary sequestration:

a) 75-85% of bronchopulmonary sequestrations are of extralobular type
b) Usually presents within the first 6 months of life
c) 40-50% are associated with congenital anomalies
d) It is commoner in the lower lobes
e) It usually communicates with the bronchial tree

26 The following statements regarding malignant mesothelioma are true:

a) Crocidolite asbestos fibres are of greater carcinogenic potential than chrysotile fibres
b) 5-10% of asbestos workers develop malignant mesothelioma in their lifetime
c) Pleural effusions are rarely associated
d) Metastases to the ipsilateral lung are seen in 50-60%
e) It predominantly involves the visceral pleura

27 Concerning mycetomas:

a) Mycetomas are fungus balls of *Aspergillus* hyphae
b) They are commonly found in the lower lobes
c) Calcification of the mycetoma occurs in over 80% of cases
d) Haemoptysis is the most important complication
e) Appearance of a crescent of air between the wall of the cavity and fungus ball is specific for mycetoma

28 The following statements regarding *Mycoplasma pneumoniae* are true:

a) It has an incubation period of 10-20 days
b) Pleural effusions are seen in 70-80%
c) Bronchiectasis is a recognised pulmonary complication
d) Mediastinal lymphadenopathy is more commonly seen in adults than children
e) The radiographic pattern is unilateral upper lobe consolidation

29 Regarding pulmonary metastases:

a) On CT imaging, haematogenous metastases are usually seen centrally in the lungs rather than peripherally
b) Cavitation is more often seen in adenocarcinoma metastases
c) Calcification is seen in chondrosarcoma metastases
d) Osteosarcoma is a recognised primary for metastases which double in size in less than 30 days
e) Thyroid carcinoma is a recognised cause of miliary metastases

30 The following statements regarding radiation pneumonitis are true:

a) Radiographic changes are seen following a radiation dose of 15 Gray
b) Adriamycin has a protective effect on the lung in reducing the reaction to radiation
c) In the acute phase, radiation pneumonitis can present with cough and pyrexia at 6-12 weeks
d) Initial radiographic changes are of localised interstitial oedema
e) Pleural effusions are a feature

31 Causes of unilateral pulmonary oedema on the side of the underlying pathology include:

a) Pulmonary contusion
b) Rapid thoracocentesis
c) Lobectomy
d) Pulmonary embolism
e) Congenital hypoplasia of the pulmonary artery

32 The following statements regarding bronchiectasis are true:

a) A 'tram line' appearance due to bronchial wall thickening and dilatation is a plain radiograph sign
b) Allergic bronchopulmonary aspergillosis is a recognised cause
c) Varicose bronchiectasis is the commonest subtype
d) Cystic bronchiectasis is associated with severe bronchial infections
e) The upper lobes are predominantly affected

33 The following statements regarding sarcoidosis are true:

a) Lymph node enlargement is seen in 80-90% of cases
b) Predominant appearance is of a mid-zone reticulonodular pattern
c) Pleural effusion is seen in 70-80%
d) Mycetoma is a common complication of advanced sarcoidosis
e) A radionuclide gallium scan can be used to assess disease activity

34 The following statements regarding alveolar cell carcinoma are true:

a) It is usually located subpleurally
b) Growth is rapid
c) It is associated with underlying pre-existing lung fibrosis
d) The diffuse pneumonic form is commoner than the local mass form
e) Air bronchograms are a feature of both forms

35 The following chest X-ray signs are associated with the following collapsed lobes:

a) Depressed horizontal fissure - right upper lobe collapse
b) Indistinct left heart border - lingular collapse
c) Horizontal orientation of the right main bronchus - right upper lobe collapse
d) Indistinct right hemidiaphragm - right lower lobe collapse
e) Right hilar elevation - right upper lobe collapse

36 Concerning traumatic aortic rupture:

a) 80-90% occur just proximal to the origin of the left subclavian artery
b) Chest X-ray features include filling in of the aortopulmonary window
c) Pseudoaneurysm is a direct sign of aortic rupture on CT
d) Widening of the right paratracheal stripe is a recognised sign
e) A normal chest X-ray is highly sensitive in excluding aortic rupture

37 The following features are more associated with *Streptococcus pneumoniae* infection rather than *Staphylococcus aureus*:

a) Cavitation
b) Empyema
c) Incidence in patients with infective endocarditis
d) Pneumatocoeles
e) Air bronchograms

38 The following statements regarding lymphangitis carcinomatosis are true:

a) It is associated with gastric cancer
b) Chest X-ray appearances are of multiple reticulonodular opacities
c) Kerley A and B lines are seen
d) Radiological changes usually precede symptom onset
e) Hilar adenopathy is seen in 80-90%

39 Regarding extrinsic allergic alveolitis:

a) It occurs in highly atopic patients
b) Acute presentation on chest X-ray is of diffuse air space consolidation
c) Is a cause of lower lobe fibrosis
d) Pleural effusions are rare in chronic extrinsic allergic alveolitis
e) Septal lines are seen in acute extrinsic allergic alveolitis

40 Features of alveolar proteinosis include:

a) 'Bat wing' air space shadowing
b) Pleural effusion
c) Lymphadenopathy
d) Cardiomegaly
e) Interstitial shadowing with Kerley B lines

1 a) True
b) True
c) True
d) True
e) True

Radiology Review Manual. 5th edition. Dahnert. Lippincott, Williams and Wilkins, 2003: 587.

2 a) False
b) True
c) True
d) False
e) False

Physics for Medical Imaging. Farr, Allisy-Roberts. Bailliere Tindell, 1996: 215-51.

3 a) False - dilatation of the pulmonary trunk
b) False - pruning of peripheral pulmonary arteries
c) True - degree of enlargement is proportionate to volume overload
d) False - condition is characterised by high pulmonary vascular resistance
e) True

Radiology Review Manual. 5th edition. Dahnert. Lippincott, Williams and Wilkins, 2003: 627-8.

4 a) True
b) False - there is a high risk of particulate emboli passing through into systemic vessels causing cerebral/myocardial infarcts. Only detachable balloons/coils are used
c) True
d) False - reduction in size with successful embolisation
e) True

Diagnostic Radiology. A Textbook of Medical Imaging. 4th edition. Grainger and Allison. Churchill Livingstone, 2001: 613.

5 a) False - 201Thallium
b) True
c) True
d) False - imaging begins 5-10 minutes after injection and completed by 30 minutes
e) False - 6 hours

Diagnostic Radiology. A Textbook of Medical Imaging. 4th edition. Grainger and Allison. Churchill Livingstone, 2001: 722-3.

6 a) False - passes above the right main bronchus
b) False - passes between the oesophagus and the trachea
c) True
d) False - causes deviation of the trachea to the left
e) False - low left hilum

Radiology Review Manual. 5th edition. Dahnert. Lippincott, Williams and Wilkins, 2003: 603.

7 a) False - approximately 8 years
b) False - Takayasu's arteritis affects main aortic branches and pulmonary arteries. External carotid artery branches are most commonly affected in temporal arteritis
c) True
d) True
e) True - with increased flow velocity and turbulence seen on US Doppler

Radiology Review Manual. 5th edition. Dahnert. Lippincott, Williams and Wilkins, 2003: 648-9.

8 a) True - thickness of the pericardium >4mm is abnormal
b) True
c) True - Kussmaul's sign
d) False - curvature of the interventricular septum to the left
e) True

Wang, *et al.* CT and MR Imaging of Pericardial Disease. *RadioGraphics* 2003; 23: 167-80.

9 a) False - left atrium
b) True - majority are sporadic
c) False - markedly hyperintense on T2, iso-hypointense on T1 weighted images
d) False - most common benign primary tumour
e) False - majority show heterogenous contrast enhancement on CT due to necrosis, cyst formation and haemorrhage

Grebeve, *et al.* Cardiac Myxoma: Imaging Features in 83 Patients. *RadioGraphics* 2002; 22: 673-87.

10 a) False - complete resolution of haematoma by 2-3 months
b) True - disappears by 3-4 weeks
c) True
d) True - suggests a fistula
e) True

Radiology Review Manual. 5th edition. Dahnert. Lippincott, Williams and Wilkins, 2003: 610.

11 a) False - 50% congenital heart disease incidence in asplenia syndrome
b) True
c) True
d) False - this is a feature of asplenia syndrome
e) True

Radiology Review Manual. 5th edition. Dahnert. Lippincott, Williams and Wilkins, 2003: 630-2.

12 a) False
b) False - bronchogenic carcinoma in 30%, breast in 7%
c) False - haematogenous spread
d) False - high signal intensity lesions on T1 weighted MRI images
e) True

Chiles, *et al.* Metastatic Involvement of Heart and Pericardium: CT and MR imaging. *RadioGraphics* 2001; 21: 439-49.

13
a) True - deep to the vein
b) True - true aneurysms of the popliteal artery are the commonest peripheral artery aneurysms
c) False - bilateral in 50-70%. Abdominal aortic aneurysm is present in 30-50% of patients with popliteal artery aneurysm
d) False - young men
e) False - there is no role for angioplasty or stenting. Surgical release of muscles/tendons causing entrapment is the treatment. Artery bypass is performed if there is thrombus/fibrosis due to chronic entrapment

Wright, *et al.* Popliteal Artery Disease: Diagnosis and Treatment. *RadioGraphics* 2004; 24: 467-8.

14
a) True
b) True
c) True
d) True
e) True - rare

Stanson, *et al.* Polyarteritis Nodosa: Spectrum of Angiographic Findings. *RadioGraphics* 2001; 21: 151-9.

15
a) True
b) False - 100 times more events are detected
c) True
d) True - with an accuracy of 92%
e) True

Rohren, *et al.* Clinical Applications of PET in Oncology. *Radiographics* 2004; 231: 305-32.

16
a) False - the commonest complication is leak of blood into the aneurysm sac (endoleak)
b) False - Type 3 endoleak arises due to defects of the graft such as a hole/laceration of graft. Type 2 endoleak involves retograde flow into the aneurysm sac via patent arteries
c) False - Type 1 endoleak is the commonest type. This involves proximal/distal leakage of blood due to incomplete graft fixation
d) False - more frequently
e) True

Mita, *et al.* Complications of Endovascular Repair for Thoracic and Abdominal Aortic Aneurysm: an Imaging Spectrum. *RadioGraphics* 2000; 20: 1263-78.

17 a) True - 15-25% of patients with myasthenia gravis have thymoma
b) True - 5% of patients with hypogammaglobulinaemia have thymoma
c) False - rare. 50% are asymptomatic
d) False - adults. 70% present in the 5-6th decade
e) True

Radiology Review Manual. 5th edition. Dahnert. Lippincott, Williams and Wilkins, 2003: 530-1.

18 a) True
b) True - though very rare
c) True
d) True
e) True

Radiology Review Manual. 5th edition. Dahnert. Lippincott, Williams and Wilkins, 2003: 583-5.
Diagnostic Radiology. A Textbook of Medical Imaging. 4th edition. Grainger and Allison. Churchill Livingstone, 2001: 845.

19 a) False - 1 end hole and 0 side holes
b) True
c) True
d) False - supine
e) False - the inferior mesenteric artery should be examined first so that contrast medium accumulation in the bladder doesn't obscure the terminal branches

A Guide to Radiological Procedures. 4th edition. Chapman and Nakielny. W.B. Saunders, 2001: 83-5.

20 a) False - cause of dilated cardiomyopathy
b) False - cause of restrictive cardiomyopathy
c) False - autosomal dominant inheritence
d) False - mitral regurgitation
e) False - global 4 chamber enlargement

Radiology Review Manual. 5th edition. Dahnert. Lippincott, Williams and Wilkins, 2003: 621-2.

21 a) True
b) True
c) False
d) False - the minor fissure is absent in 10%
e) False - the mid-axillary line

Anatomy for Diagnostic Imaging. 2nd edition. Ryan, McNichols and Eustace. W.B. Saunders, 2004; Chapter 4: 118-9.

22 a) False
b) True
c) True
d) False
e) True

Radiology Review Manual. 5th edition. Dahnert. Lippincott, Williams and Wilkins, 2003: 574-5.

23 a) True
b) False - posterior
c) True
d) True
e) False - right lateral relationship

Anatomy for Dagnostic Imaging. 2nd edition. Ryan, McNichols and Eustace. W.B. Saunders, 2004; Chapter 4: 116-7.

24 a) True
b) False - upper and lower zones of relatively normal calibre aorta of at least 15mm is required though 20mm is preferable
c) True
d) False - it is suitable for descending but not ascending thoracic aortic aneurysms
e) True - this reduces the risk of the stent slipping

Morgan. Endovascular Management of Diseases of the Thoracic Aorta. *Radiology Now* 2004; 21: 2.

25 a) False - 75% are intralobular
b) True
c) True
d) True
e) False - no communication with the bronchial tree

Radiology Review Manual. 5th edition. Dahnert. Lippincott, Williams and Wilkins, 2003: 471-2.

26 a) True
b) True - there is a latent peiod of 20-40 years
c) False - 70-80% have pleural effusions
d) True
e) False - parietal pleura

Muller, *et al.* Imaging of the Pleura. *Radiology* 1993; 186: 297.

27 a) True
b) False - upper lobes and the superior segments of the lower lobes. Most commonly found in TB cavities
c) False - rare
d) True - sometimes haemorrhage is so severe that surgical resection is required
e) False - similar appearance can be seen with a hydatid and cavitatory neoplasm

Diagnostic Radiology. A Textbook of Medical Imaging. 4th edition. Grainger and Allison. Churchill Livingstone, 2001: 398-9.

28 a) True
b) False - rare
c) True
d) False - commoner in children
e) False - lower lobes are involved. Multilobar and bilateral disease are also observed

Diagnostic Radiology. A Textbook of Medical Imaging. 4th edition. Grainger and Allison. Churchill Livingstone, 2001: 384-5.

29 a) False - haematogenous metastases are peripheral
b) False - cavitation is more often seen in squamous cell carcinoma metastases
c) True
d) True - also observed with choriocarcinoma metastases
e) True - causes of miliary metastases include renal cell carcinoma, bone sarcomas and choriocarcinoma

Diagnostic Radiology. A Textbook of Medical Imaging. 4th edition. Grainger and Allison. Churchill Livingstone, 2001: 482-5.

30 a) False - clinical and radiological changes are not seen with doses of <20 Gray. Most have changes following a dose of 40 Gray.
b) False - chemotherapeutic agents, e.g. Adriamycin, Bleomycin and Cyclophosphamide potentiate the effect. Pneumonitis presents earlier and is more severe
c) True
d) True - can progress to airspace consolidation and atelectasis
e) True - but not common

Diagnostic Radiology. A Textbook of Medical Imaging. 4th edition. Grainger and Allison. Churchill Livingstone, 2001: 559-60.

31 a) True
b) True
c) False - contralateral side
d) False - contralateral side
e) False - contralateral side

Radiology Review Manual. 5th edition. Dahnert. Lippincott, Williams and Wilkins, 2003: 265.

32 a) True
b) True
c) False - varicose bronchiectasis is rare. Associated with Swyer-James syndrome. Cylindrical bronchiectasis is the commonest subtype
d) True
e) False - posterobasal segments of the lower lobes

Radiology Review Manual. 5th edition. Dahnert. Lippincott, Williams and Wilkins, 2003: 464.

33 a) True
b) True
c) False - pleural effusion is seen in 2-3%
d) True - chronic advanced disease can cause progressive fibrosis, lung retraction and bullae formation
e) True - uptake in salivary glands, lymph nodes and lung parenchyma is correlated with disease activity

Koyama, *et al.* Radiologic Manifestations of Sarcoidosis in Various Organs. *RadioGraphics* 2004; 24: 87.

34 a) True
b) False - doubling time is longer than 18 months
c) True - associated with pre-existing pulmonary scarring and scleroderma
d) False - diffuse pneumonic form accounts for 10-40%
e) True

Radiology Review Manual. 5th edition. Dahnert. Lippincott, Williams and Wilkins, 2003: 466-7.
Diagnostic Radiology. A Textbook of Medical Imaging. 4th edition. Grainger and Allison. Churchill Livingstone, 2001: 469-70.

35 a) False - middle lobe collapse
b) True
c) True
d) True
e) True

Diagnostic Radiology. A Textbook of Medical Imaging. 4th edition. Grainger and Allison. Churchill Livingstone, 2001: 438-41.

36 a) False - 80-90% occur just distal to the origin of the left subclavian artery
b) True - this is a sign of mediastinal haematoma
c) True
d) True
e) True - a normal chest radiograph has a negative predictive value of 96-98%

Diagnostic Radiology. A Textbook of Medical Imaging. 4th edition. Grainger and Allison. Churchill Livingstone, 2001: 540-1.

37 a) False
b) False
c) False
d) False
e) True

Diagnostic Radiology. A Textbook of Medical Imaging. 4th edition. Grainger and Allison. Churchill Livingstone, 2001: 378-80.

38 a) True - associated with cancer of the cervix, colon, stomach, breast, pancreas, thyroid and larynx
b) True
c) True - sign of lymphatic obstruction
d) False - shortness of breath precedes chest X-ray changes
e) False - hilar adenopathy is seen in 20-50%

Radiology Review Manual. 5th edition. Dahnert. Lippincott, Williams and Wilkins, 2003: 502.

39 a) False - occurs in non-atopic patients as a response to organic dusts
b) True
c) False - upper lobe fibrosis
d) True
e) True

Radiology Review Manual. 5th edition. Dahnert. Lippincott, Williams and Wilkins, 2003: 486-7.

40 a) True
b) False
c) False
d) False
e) True - chronic stage

Godwin, *et al.* Pulmonary Alveolar Proteinosis: CT Findings. *Radiology* 1988; 169: 609.

Paper 2
Musculoskeletal and Trauma

1 Morton neuroma:
a) Is typically found in the 4th intermetatarsal space
b) Is of high signal on T2 weighted MRI
c) Is asymptomatic
d) On ultrasound, has the appearance of an ovoid hypoechoic mass orientated parallel to the long axis of the metatarsal bones
e) Has a high malignant potential

2 The following are recognised associations:
a) Madelung's deformity and Turner's syndrome
b) Superior rib notching and osteogenesis imperfecta
c) Erosion of the outer end of the clavicle and pyknodysostosis
d) Erlenmeyer flask deformity and Noonan's syndrome
e) Arachnodactyly and homocystinuria

3 Causes of acro-osteolysis include:
a) Leprosy
b) Frostbite
c) Hyperparathyroidism
d) Phenytoin toxicity
e) Syringomyelia

4 The following statements regarding bone marrow are true:
a) Yellow marrow decreases with age
b) Red marrow is of high signal on T1 weighted MRI images
c) Yellow marrow is of high signal on T2 weighted MRI images
d) Radiotherapy causes marked reduction in yellow marrow
e) Osteopetrosis is characterised by reduced signal on T2 weighted MRI images

5 Concerning aneurysmal bone cysts:

a) 60-80% of aneurysmal bone cysts are found in under 20-year-olds
b) Periosteal reaction is a pathognomonic feature
c) Hypervascularity is usually seen in the periphery of the lesion
d) They demonstrate a fluid-fluid level on CT
e) They have a recurrence rate of 20-30% after surgical treatment

6 Regarding blunt trauma to the pancreas:

a) Injury to the pancreas occurs in 25-30% of blunt abdominal trauma patients
b) The majority of injuries occur in the pancreatic tail
c) Isolated pancreatic injuries occur in 85-90% of cases
d) A pancreatic laceration appears as a high attenuation lesion on contrast-enhanced CT
e) Integrity of the pancreatic duct is an important factor in determining outcome following pancreatic injury

7 Shoulder anatomy:

a) In an intact rotator cuff there is communication between the glenohumeral joint and the subacromial-subdeltoid bursae
b) Subscapularis, infraspinatus and teres minor insert onto the greater tuberosity
c) Rotator cuff tears most commonly involve the supraspinatus portion of the cuff
d) Long head of biceps runs in the bicipital groove to insert into the infraglenoid tubercle
e) Normal glenoid labrum is of high signal on a T2 weighted fat-saturated MRI image

8 Desirable properties of a radionuclide for imaging are:

a) Decay to a stable daughter
b) A physical half-life of a few minutes
c) Decay by electron capture
d) Decay by isomeric transition
e) Emit gamma rays of energy 350-550 kiloelectronvolts (keV)

9 Regarding diffuse idiopathic skeletal hyperostosis:

a) Highest incidence in the 3rd to 5th decades
b) Most commonly involves the cervical spine
c) Sacroiliac joints are usually involved when the lumbar spine is
d) Extraspinal ligamentous hyperostosis is a feature
e) In the thoracic spine the hyperostotic changes are more prominent on the right

10 Vertebroplasty:

a) Has no role in patients with osteolytic vertebral metastases
b) Use of percutaneous vertebroplasty in patients with multiple myeloma prevents subsequent radiation therapy
c) Extensive vertebral destruction is a contraindication to vertebroplasty
d) For the lumbar spine, a 12-15-gauge needle is used
e) Methyl methacrylate polymer cement is used

11 The following descriptions of the fractures are correct:

a) Monteggia fracture - ulnar fracture with dislocation of the radial head
b) Galleazi fracture - distal radial fracture with dislocation of distal radioulnar joint
c) Segond fracture - cortical avulsion fracture of proximal lateral tibia
d) Chauffer's fracture - triangular fracture of radial styloid process
e) Pott's fracture - tibia fracture above an intact tibiofibular ligament

12 Trauma to the spleen:

a) In blunt abdominal trauma the spleen is injured in 50-60% of significant abdominal injuries
b) Hypotension is a presenting symptom of splenic trauma in less than 40% of cases
c) At least 500ml of intra-abdominal fluid is required for detection by focused abdominal ultrasonography in trauma (FAST)
d) Splenic injury can be reliably excluded by the absence of free fluid in the peritoneal cavity
e) Acute splenic lacerations appear as hyperechoic regions on ultrasound

13 Regarding lumbar spondylolisthesis:

a) Degenerative spondylolisthesis most commonly affects L5/S1
b) Spondyloptosis is a complete slip of L5 on S1
c) Degenerative spondylolisthesis is commoner in men
d) Facet joint synovial cysts are associated with degenerative spondylolisthesis
e) Traumatic spondylolisthesis accounts for 20-30% of spondylolistheses

14 Causes for a superscan on bone scintigraphy include:

a) Renal osteodystrophy
b) Osteomalacia
c) Hyperparathyroidism
d) Hyperthyroidism
e) Diffuse skeletal metastases

15 The following are features of hypervitaminosis D:

a) Increased density of the skull
b) Widened zone of provisional calcification
c) Soft tissue calcification
d) Osteoporosis
e) Nephrocalcinosis

16 Features of rheumatoid arthritis include:

a) Late involvement of the 2nd and 3rd metacarpophalangeal joints
b) Central bone erosions
c) Ulnar subluxation
d) Juxta-articular osteoporosis
e) Calcification of the triangular fibrocartilage complex

17 The following are skeletal features of tuberous sclerosis:

a) Multiple bone islands
b) Periosteal reactions
c) Cystic bone lesions
d) Rib expansion
e) Multiple non-ossifying fibromas

18 **The following statements regarding Sudeck's dystrophy are true:**

a) It affects 5-10% of all trauma patients
b) Plain radiograph appearances are of patchy osteopaenia
c) Have increased uptake on a 3-phase bone scan
d) It is associated with Raynaud's phenomenon
e) Atrophy of the soft tissues occurs early

19 **The following are features of Gaucher's disease:**

a) Generalised osteopaenia
b) Marked cortical thickening
c) Endosteal scalloping
d) Biconcave 'fish-mouth' vertebrae
e) Madelung's deformity

20 **Regarding stress fractures:**

a) 16-detector multislice CT is more accurate than skeletal scintigraphy at identifying stress fractures
b) Stress fractures account for less than 1% of all significant sporting injuries
c) A stress fracture is characterised by reduced uptake at the fracture site on a 99m technetium MDP bone scan
d) Stress fractures only occur in an osteoporotic skeleton
e) Zwas' system consists of criteria used for diagnosing stress fractures

21 **Features found in pigmented villonodular synovitis:**

a) Predominantly polyarticular distribution
b) Haemorrhagic 'chocolate' effusion
c) Calcification in 50-60%
d) Joint space narrowing is early
e) MRI appearances of high signal on T1 weighted spin-echo MRI images

22 Regarding arthrography:

a) 10ml of air is appropriate for a double-contrast knee arthrogram in an adult
b) Perthes' disease is an indication for hip arthrography
c) A 22-gauge lumbar puncture needle is commonly used for shoulder arthrography
d) In ankle arthrography 6-8ml of LOCM 240 is used
e) Presence of intra-articular loose bodies are a recognised contraindication to knee arthrography

23 The following statements regarding musculoskeletal MRI are true:

a) A surface coil gives an improved resolution than the body coil
b) Gradient echo sequences can differentiate articular cartilage from effusion
c) A total hip replacement is usually an absolute contraindication to MRI
d) T wave elevation on ECG is a recognised physiological change by the static magnetic field of the MRI scanner
e) Claustrophobia may occur in as many as 20% of patients

24 Regarding imaging appearances of osteomyelitis:

a) Radiographic findings become evident approximately 3 days after onset of infection
b) Periosteal reaction is the earliest sign of acute osteomyelitis
c) Klebsiella is the commonest organism isolated in adults
d) Chronic osteomyelitis is characterised by prominent cortical thinning
e) The diaphyses are often spared in patients with sickle cell disease

25 The following statements regarding the imaging of acute cervical spine injuries are true:

a) 10-20% of significant cervical spine injuries are not identified on plain radiographs
b) Flexion/extension views are of little use in the acute setting
c) CT is the imaging modality of choice for soft tissue injuries
d) A fall of greater than 3 metres is a high risk parameter for cervical spine injury
e) T2 fat-saturated images are useful in assessing for bone marrow oedema

26 The following are causes of painful sclerosis of the medial end of the clavicle:

a) Osteoarthritis
b) Sternoclavicular pyoarthrosis
c) Condensing osteitis
d) Sternocostoclavicular hyperostosis
e) Freidrich's disease

27 Regarding imaging of periosteal reactions:

a) Periosteal reaction becomes apparent 10-20 days following insult
b) Single layered periosteal reaction is a physiological appearance in premature infants
c) Osteomyelitis is a recognised cause of solid periosteal reaction
d) Sunburst periosteal reaction is seen in relation to aggressive tumours
e) Aggressive malignant primary bone tumours are a cause of Codman's triangle

28 Regarding trauma:

a) Salter Harris 2 fractures involve the articular surface
b) A posterior fat pad can be a normal finding on a lateral X-ray of the elbow
c) Avulsion of the flexor tendon results in a mallet finger
d) Tracking Mcgregor's line 1 will help to identify a fracture through the inferior orbital rim
e) In a fracture of the 5th metatarsal the fracture line is usually longitudinal to the long axis of the metatarsal

29 The following statements regarding a burst fracture of a vertebral body are true:

a) This is most commonly associated with a shearing injury
b) It is most commonly found from T4-T8
c) Other spinal injuries are associated in up to 10-15% of cases
d) Reduced interpedicular distance is a sign on an AP film
e) Concavity of the posterior cortical line is a sign on lateral film

30 The following are features of transient osteoporosis of the hip:

a) Usually painless
b) Joint space narrowing
c) Reduced uptake on bone scan
d) Pathological fractures are rare
e) Usually bilateral and symmetrical

1 a) False - 3rd intermetatarsal space
b) False - low
c) False - usually presents with burning/electric forefoot pain
d) False - hyperechoic
e) False - benign lesion

Diagnosis of Bone and Joint Disorders. 4th edition. Resnick. W.B. Saunders, 2002: 3533.

2 a) True - other causes include diaphyseal aclasia, post-infection, post-trauma, Leri-Weil disease
b) True - other causes include rheumatoid arthritis, systemic lupus erythematosus, scleroderma, Sjögren's disease, hyperparathyroidism, neurofibromatosis, poliomyelitis, progeria, Marfan's syndrome
c) True - other causes include rheumatoid arthritis, multiple myeloma, metastases, hyperparathyroidism, cleidocranial dysplasia
d) False
e) True - Marfan's syndrome is another cause

Radiology Review Manual. 5th edition. Dahnert. Lippincott, Williams and Wilkins, 2003: 2-172.

3 a) True
b) True
c) True
d) True
e) True

Aids to Radiological Differential Diagnosis. 4th edition. Chapman and Nakielny. W.B. Saunders, 2003: 60-1.

4 a) False - yellow marrow increases with age
b) False - red marrow is of low signal on T1 and high signal on T2 weighted MRI images
c) True - yellow marrow is of high signal on T1 and T2 weighted MRI images
d) False
e) True - osteopetrosis is characterised by reduced signal on T1 and T2 weighted MRI images

Aids to Radiological Differential Diagnosis. 4th edition. Chapman and Nakielny. W.B. Saunders, 2003: 64.

5 a) True
b) False - no periosteal reaction unless there is a fracture
c) True - peripheral hypervascularity is seen in 75% of lesions
d) True
e) True - recurrence rate of 20-30%

Radiology Review Manual. 5th edition. Dahnert. Lippincott, Williams and Wilkins, 2003: 43.

6 a) False - pancreatic injury occurs in 2%
b) False - two thirds of injuries occur in the pancreatic body
c) False - 90% of cases have associated injuries, especially to the liver, spleen, duodenum and stomach
d) False - low attenuation lesion
e) True - pancreatic duct disruption is associated with increased fistula and abscess formation, and increased mortality

Gupta *et al.* Blunt Trauma of the Pancreas and Biliary Tract: a Multimodality Imaging Approach to Diagnosis. *RadioGraphics* 2004; 24: 1381-95.

7 a) False - no communication
b) False - supraspinatus, infraspinatus and teres minor attach to the greater trochanter, subscapularis attaches to the lesser tuberosity
c) True
d) False - supraglenoid tubercle
e) False - low signal

Orthopaedic Radiology - a Practical Approach. 2nd edition. Greenspan. Raven Press, 1992; Chapter 5: Shoulder.

8 a) True
b) False - if too short, much more activity must be prepared than is actually injected. Therefore, a half-life of a few hours is preferred
c) True
d) True
e) False - 50-300 keV

Physics for Medical Imaging. Farr, Allisy-Roberts. Bailliere Tindell, 1996: 135-6.

9
a) False - >50years. Males. Females
b) False - lower thoracic spine
c) False - no sacroiliac joint involvement though sometimes appearances in the spine are similar to ankylosing spondylitis
d) True - most often seen at the pelvis, patella, calcaneum, olecranon
e) True - pulsating aorta on left side reduces ossification

Diagnostic Radiology. A Textbook of Medical Imaging. 4th edition. Grainger and Allison. Churchill Livingstone, 2001: 863-5.

10
a) False - common indications are metastases, osteoporotic collapse, vertebral haemangiomas
b) False - radiation has no effect on the constitution of cement
c) False - significant destruction/collapse makes the procedure difficult but not a contraindication. Contraindications include infection, coagulation disorders, if facilities for emergency decompression surgery are not available
d) False - lumbar and lower thoracic - 10-11-gauge, cervical and upper thoracic - 12-15-gauge
e) True

Silva, Cotten. Vertebroplasty. *Radiology Now* 2002; 19 (2): 14-8.

11
a) True
b) True
c) True
d) True
e) False - fibula fracture

Radiology Review Manual. 5th edition. Dahnert. Lippincott, Williams and Wilkins, 2003: 84-8.

12
a) False - 20-30%
b) True - 25-30%
c) False - about 100mls
d) False - 12% have no free fluid
e) False - hypoechoic lesion

Doody, *et al.* Blunt Trauma to the Spleen, US Findings. *Clinical Radiology* 2005; 60 (9): 968-76.

13 a) False - L4/5
b) True
c) False - 4 times more in women
d) True
e) False - rare

Yi, *et al.* The Imaging of Lumbar Spondylolisthesis. *Clinical Radiology* 2005; 60 (5): 543-6.

14 a) True
b) True
c) True
d) True
e) True

Radiology Review Manual. 5th edition. Dahnert. Lippincott, Williams and Wilkins, 2003: 1080-1.

15 a) True
b) True
c) True
d) True - late feature
e) True

Aids to Radiological Differential Diagnosis. 4th edition. Chapman and Nakielny. W.B. Saunders, 2003: 10.

16 a) False
b) True - marginal and central erosions
c) True
d) True
e) False

Radiology Review Manual. 5th edition. Dahnert. Lippincott, Williams and Wilkins, 2003: 151.

17 a) True
b) True
c) True
d) True
e) False - this is a feature in neurofibromatosis

Radiology Review Manual. 5th edition. Dahnert. Lippincott, Williams and Wilkins, 2003: 352.

18 a) False - 0.01% of all trauma patients are affected
b) True - patchy osteopaenia is seen in 50% as early as 2-3 weeks after symptom onset
c) True
d) True
e) False - this is an end-stage feature

Radiology Review Manual. 5th edition. Dahnert. Lippincott, Williams and Wilkins, 2003: 148.

19 a) True
b) False
c) True
d) True
e) False

Radiology Review Manual. 5th edition. Dahnert. Lippincott, Williams and Wilkins, 2003: 91-2.

20 a) False
b) False - account for more than 10%
c) False - increased uptake at the fracture site on 99m technetium MDP bone scan
d) False - stress fractures occur as a result of a repetitive strain on a bone that has not accommodated itself to this. Insufficience fractures occur when a normal physiologic stress is applied to abnormal bone
e) True

Groves, *et al.* 16-detector Multislice CT in the Detection of Stress Fractures: a Comparison with Skeletal Scintigraphy. *Clinical Radiology* 2005; 60 (10): 1100-5.

21 a) False - monoarticular
b) True
a) False - no calcification
b) False - joint space narrowing is a late feature
c) False - characteristic appearances of low signal on T1 and T2 weighted spin-echo MRI images due to presence of iron

Radiology Review Manual. 5th edition. Dahnert. Lippincott, Williams and Wilkins, 2003: 144.

22 a) False - 40ml of air is required
b) True - other causes include developmental dysplasia of the hip, trauma, arthropathy
c) True
d) True
e) False

A Guide to Radiological Procedures. 4th edition. Chapman and Nakielny. W.B. Saunders, 2001: 264-82.

23 a) True
b) True
c) False - most orthopaedic implants are safe
d) True
e) False - 10%, 1% of investigations are curtailed

A Guide to Radiological Procedures. 4th edition. Chapman and Nakielny. W.B. Saunders, 2001: 263-4.

24 a) False - 1-2 weeks
b) False - soft tissue swelling and loss of normal fat planes
c) False
d) False - thickening
e) False - infection focus at diaphyseal infarcts

Musculoskeletal Imaging: The Requisites. 1st edition. Sartoris. Mosby, 1996: Chapter 2.

25 a) True - due to poor radiography, errors of image interpretation and absence of signs
b) True - delayed flexion/extension views helpful in identifying soft tissue injuries
c) False - MRI
d) True
e) True - increased signal areas

Tins, Cassar-Pukkicino. Imaging of Acute Cervical Spine Injuries: Review and Outlook. *Clinical Radiology* 2004; 59 (10): 865-80.

26 a) True
b) True
c) True
d) True
e) True - other causes include sclerotic metastases, osteoid osteoma, osteosarcoma, Paget's disease and fibrous dysplasia

Harden, *et al.* Painful Sclerosis of the Medial End of the Clavicle. *Clinical Radiology* 2004; 59 (11): 992-9.

27 a) True
b) True - physiological appearance in premature infants up to 6 months old
c) True
d) True - osteosarcoma is commonest
e) True - osteomyelitis and trauma are other causes

Wenaden, *et al.* Imaging of Periosteal Reactions Associated with Focal Lesions of Bone. *Clinical Radiology* 2005; 60 (4): 439-55.

28 a) False - Salter Harris 3 and 4 are intra-articular
b) False
c) False - extensor tendons
d) False - line 2 passes through the zygomatic arch and inferior orbital rim
e) False - the fracture line is transverse to the long axis of the metatarsal

Accident and Emergency Radiology. 1st edition. Raby, Berman, de Lacy. W.B. Saunders, 1995.

29 a) False - vertical compression injury
b) False - T12-L2
c) False - other spinal injuries are associated in up to 40% of cases
d) False - increased interpedicular distance is a sign on an AP film
e) False - convexity of the posterior cortical line is a sign on lateral film

Muskuloskeletal Imaging Companion. 1st edition. Thomas H. Berquist. Lippincott, Williams and Wilkins, 2002: 70.

30 a) False
b) False
c) False - increased
d) False - common
e) False

Radiology Review Manual. 5th edition. Dahnert. Lippincott, Williams and Wilkins, 2003: 167.

Paper 3

Gastrointestinal

1 Regarding Peutz-Jeghers syndrome:

a) It is inherited in an autosomal recessive manner
b) There is an association with intussusception
c) Polyps are seen in the stomach
d) Patients are at increased risk of gastrointestinal adenocarcinoma
e) It is associated with pigmented lesions on the fingers

2 The following statements regarding familial adenomatous polyposis syndrome are true:

a) Its inheritence pattern is autosomal dominant
b) Clinical symptoms become evident during the 5th-6th decade
c) Polyps are identified in the stomach in 5% of affected cases
d) It is associated with peri-ampullary carcinoma
e) It is associated with alopecia

3 Regarding carcinoid tumour:

a) It is rarely multiple
b) Carcinoid sydrome is the presentation in only 20-30% of cases
c) The commonest location for this tumour is the appendix
d) 50% of tumours greater than 2cm in size have metastases
e) Angulation of small bowel loops on small bowel follow through is a diagnostic feature

4 The following statements regarding achalasia are correct:

a) Dilatation of the oesophagus begins in the upper third
b) Multiple non-peristaltic contractions are seen on barium swallow
c) There is an association with Plummer-Vinson syndrome
d) A prominent gastric air bubble is seen on erect CXR
e) Squamous cell carcinoma of the oesophagus is a recognised complication

5 Regarding toxic megacolon:

a) Ischaemic colitis is the most common underlying pathological cause
b) Multiple air fluid levels are seen on plain abdominal X-ray
c) Barium enema is contraindicated
d) Has a mortality of 5-8%
e) Can present as bloody diarrhoea

6 The following statements regarding lymphoma of the gastrointestinal tract are true:

a) There is an increased risk associated with ulcerative colitis
b) The stomach is the most common site of involvement by non-Hodgkin's lymphoma
c) Diffuse involvement of the whole stomach is seen in 10-15%
d) In the colon the rectum is most commonly involved
e) Presents with thickened valvulae conniventes in the small bowel

7 Duodenal ulcers:

a) Are usually associated with a normal level of gastric acid secretion
b) Are most likely to be found in the posterior wall of the duodenal bulb
c) Are usually greater than 2cm in size
d) Perforation is a complication in 20-30%
e) Vagotomy is a recognised treatment

8 Regarding oesphageal duplication cysts:

a) The oesophagus is the commonest site for duplication cysts in the alimentary canal
b) They are more commonly found on the left side
c) There is an association with spina bifida
d) 50-60% occur in the mid-oesophagus
e) On a PA CXR they can be mistaken for a hiatus hernia

9 The following features are commoner in Crohn's disease than in ulcerative colitis:

a) Toxic megacolon
b) Increased risk of colonic carcinoma
c) Formation of vesicocolic fistula
d) Thickening of the ileocaecal valve
e) Shallow ulcers

10 The following drugs reduce gastric emptying:

a) Buscopan
b) Glucagon
c) Metoclopramide
d) Procyclidine
e) Indomethacin

11 Giardiasisis is associated with:

a) Gastric varices
b) Hypoperistalsis with a reduced transit time
c) Malabsorption
d) Thickened small bowel mucosal folds
e) Ulceration

12 Regarding peritoneal spaces:

a) The right subhepatic space communicates with the lesser sac
b) The bare area of the liver is located between reflections of the right and left coronary ligaments
c) The left subphrenic space is separated from the right subphrenic space by the falciform ligament
d) The splenorenal ligament separates the left subphrenic space from the left paracolic gutter
e) The gastrocolic ligament connects the lesser curve of the stomach to the superior aspect of the transverse colon

13 Regarding CT colonography:

a) No preparation is required
b) Images are acquired with the patient supine and prone
c) A mass which does not move after changing patient position represents a polyp
d) Extracolonic findings that require further investigation are found in 10% of patients
e) The appendix orifice can be differentiated from tumour by coronal reformats

14 Imaging features of acute appendicitis include:

a) Enlarged appendix >6mm in diameter
b) Enlarged mesenteric lymph nodes
c) Presence of appendicolith
d) Focal caecal apical wall thickening
e) Peri-appendiceal fat stranding

15 Regarding gastrointestinal stromal tumours (GIST):

a) The most significant criteria for predicting malignant potential is tumour size
b) The commonest location is the sigmoid
c) It is a cause of haematemesis
d) There is an association with neurofibromatosis Type 1
e) Contrast enhancement is invariably uniform

16 Regarding MR imaging of anal cancer:

a) Anal cancer is associated with infection with human papilloma virus
b) Anal cancer is usually an adenocarcinoma
c) The dentate line of the anal canal is identified on MRI
d) Tumours arising below the dentate line spread to internal iliac lymph nodes
e) Primary anal tumours are of high signal intensity on T2 weighted images

17 Regarding small bowel obstruction:

a) Adhesions are responsible for 20-25% of small bowel obstructions
b) Right-sided paraduodenal hernias are commoner than the left
c) Adenocarcinomas of the small bowel usually arise in the ileum
d) Gas within the bowel wall is an imaging feature of a bowel infarct
e) Small bowel intussusceptions can occur in coeliac disease

18 Regarding post-transplantation lymphoproliferative disorder (PTLD):

a) It most commonly occurs in renal transplant patients
b) PTLD contributes to death in 10-12% of transplant recipients
c) Mean presentation occurs 40-50 months post-transplantation
d) Extranodal disease is considerably less common than in lymphoma affecting non-immunocompromised people
e) The spleen is the most frequently affected organ

19 Causes of disproportionate fat stranding in excess of the degree of bowel wall thickening include:

a) Crohn's disease
b) Omental infarction
c) Diverticulitis
d) Epiploic appendigitis
e) Ischaemic bowel

20 Regarding oesophageal balloon dilatation and stent placement:

a) In benign strictures, oesophageal dilatation has technical success in 90-95%
b) Oesophageal stent placement relieves dysphagia in 50-60%
c) An oesophageal stricture should be evaluated with endoscopy before dilatation/stent placement
d) Risk of perforation following dilatation is 2-3%
e) Stents are more likely to migrate proximally

21 Regarding hepatic adenoma:

a) It is associated with Type 1 glycogen storage disease
b) Is located in the left lobe of the liver in 60-75% of cases
c) Is easily differentiated from hepatocellular carcinoma on MRI
d) Is hypovasular
e) Often reduces in size during pregnancy

22 Causes of hepatic lesions with a central scar include:

a) Hepatic adenoma
b) Fibrolamellar hepatocellular carcinoma
c) Focal nodular hyperplasia
d) Giant cavernous haemangioma
e) Hepatic lymphoma

23 Features of an annular pancreas include:

a) It occurs when part of the dorsal bud fails to atrophy
b) Associated with an imperforate anus
c) Usually involves the 3rd part of the duodenum
d) The 'double-bubble' sign is seen on plain abdominal radiograph
e) There is an increased incidence of peptic ulcers

24 The following statements regarding primary sclerosing cholangitis is true:

a) It affects only the intrahepatic bile ducts
b) The common bile duct is usually spared
c) Echogenic portal triads are identified on ultrasound
d) There is a 10-15 times increased risk of developing cholangiocarcinoma
e) It is associated with positive antimitochondrial antibodies

25 Regarding fibrolamellar hepatocellular carcinoma:
a) Alcoholic cirrhosis is a recognised risk factor
b) Commonly occurs in the elderly
c) Calcification is rare
d) The central scar is hypointense on T1 and hyperintense on T2 weighted MRI images
e) Has a good prognosis

26 Features of primary biliary cirrhosis include:
a) Xanthelasma
b) Involvement of the intra and extrahepatic bile ducts
c) Prolongation of hepatic Tc-99m IDA clearance
d) Non-visualisation of the gallbladder on oral cholecystogram
e) Affects 30-50-year-old women

27 Gastrointestinal features of cystic fibrosis include:
a) Portal hypertension
b) Mega-gallbladder
c) Lipomatous pseudohypertrophy of the pancreas
d) Increased calibre of colon
e) Meconium ileus

28 With respect to technetium 99m sulphur colloid scan:
a) Imaging is performed 60 minutes post-IV injection of radioisotope
b) 85% of the radioisotope accumulates in the liver
c) In Budd-Chiari syndrome the caudate lobe has relative increased uptake of radioisotope
d) Colloid shift away from the liver is seen with long-term corticosteroid therapy
e) Regenerating nodules of cirrhosis appear as focal 'cold' liver lesions

29 The following statements regarding cavernous haemangioma of the liver are true:

a) Most lesions are >5cm in size
b) They appear uniformly hypoechoic on ultrasound
c) Are of high signal intensity on T2 weighted MRI images
d) Arteriovenous shunts supplying them are identified on hepatic angiography
e) Contrast enhancement on CT usually lasts for only 3 minutes due to rapid flow

30 The following are true of gallbladder carcinoma:

a) Cholelithiasis is seen in 70-80% of patients with gallbladder carcinoma
b) On ultrasound, diffuse thickening of the gallbladder wall may be found
c) The body of the gallbladder is the commonest site
d) A haematogenous route is the most likely mode of spread
e) Most are squamous cell carcinomas

31 Regarding pancreatic anatomy:

a) It lies at the level of L3
b) Lies anterior to the splenic vein
c) A main duct measuring 5mm in diameter is within normal limits
d) The superior pancreaticoduodenal artery is a branch of the superior mesenteric artery
e) The accessory duct drains into the duodenum 2cm distal to the main duct

32 The following statements regarding percutaneous transhepatic cholangiography are true:

a) Hydatid disease is a contraindication
b) A 22-gauge Chiba needle is used
c) No patient preparation is required
d) Access is gained at the right mid-clavicular line
e) If a duct is not entered after 4 attempts, the procedure is terminated

33 Regarding ultrasound of the gallbladder:

a) Patient preparation with fasting for at least 6 hours is advised
b) A 3-5 MHz ultrasound transducer is used
c) A normal gallbladder wall measures <3mm
d) An internal diameter measurement of the adult common hepatic duct of 8mm is within normal limits
e) The common bile duct lies anterior to the hepatic artery in 15-20%

34 The following are causes of fatty replacement of the pancreas:

a) Diabetes mellitus
b) Haemochromatosis
c) Chronic pancreatitis
d) Cushing's disease
e) Malnutrition

35 Regarding splenic angiosarcoma:

a) Is the most common primary neoplasm of the spleen
b) Is associated with toxic exposure to vinyl chloride
c) 70% metastasise to the liver
d) Most commonly found in adults >70 years of age
e) Spontaneous rupture occurs in one third of cases

36 The following statements regarding emphysematous cholecystitis are true:

a) There is a predisposition in diabetics
b) *Clostridium perfringens* is a recognised causative organism
c) The white cell count is rarely elevated
d) Gas appears 4-5 days after onset of symptoms
e) Pneumobilia is a common sign on plain film

37 Imaging features of a failure of a transjugular intrahepatic portosystemic shunt (TIPS) are:

a) Shunt velocity of 90cm/s
b) Retrograde flow in the right hepatic vein
c) Increased pulsatility of portal flow
d) Reversal of portal venous flow direction
e) Developing ascites

38 Imaging features of cirrhosis of the liver include:

a) Hypertrophy of the lateral segment of the left lobe
b) Increased hepatic parenchymal echogenicity on ultrasound
c) Dampened oscillations of the hepatic vein on Doppler ultrasound
d) Regenerating nodules are of reduced intensity on T2 weighted MRI images
e) Constriction of hepatic arteries

39 The following statements regarding the anatomy of the oesophagus are true:

a) It pierces the diaphragm at level of T10
b) The lower third is supplied by the right gastric artery
c) The aberrant right subclavian artery passes anterior to the oesophagus
d) The Z line identifies the squamocolumnar junction
e) The oesophageal mucosa is angled in longitudinal folds which normally measure 3-4mm thickness

40 The following are causes of colonic thumbprinting:

a) Ulcerative colitis
b) Behcet's disease
c) Cytomegalovirus in renal transplant patients
d) Pseudomembranous colitis
e) Lymphoma

1 a) False - autosomal dominant
b) True
c) True - polyps are usually in the small bowel, most commonly seen in the jejunum but polyps are also seen in the colon and stomach
d) True - but polyps themselves are hamartomatous polyps and are benign
e) True - multiple melanin spots are seen on mucous membranes, facial skin, fingers and toes

Fundamentals of Diagnostic Radiology. 2nd edition. Brant and Helms. Lippincott, Williams and Wilkins, 1999: 741.

2 a) True
b) False - usually presents 20-30-year-olds
c) True
d) True
e) False - small bowel polyps, nail atrophy, brown skin pigmentation and alopecia are features of Canada-Cronkhite syndrome

Fundamentals of Diagnostic Radiology. 2nd edition. Brant and Helms. Lippincott, Williams and Wilkins, 1999: 754-5.

3 a) False - 33% are multiple
b) False - carcinoid sydrome is the presentation in 7% of cases. Syndrome arises due to excess serotonin levels
c) True - located in the appendix in 30-45%
d) False - 50% of tumours of 1-2cm in size have metastases, 85% of tumours greater than 2cm have metastases
e) True - there is a strong desmoplastic response in the mesentery, resulting in angulation and kinking of small bowel loops which can cause small bowel obstruction

Radiology Review Manual. 5th edition. Dahnert. Lippincott, Williams and Wilkins, 2003: 801-2.

4 a) True - progresses to involve the entire length
b) True
c) False
d) False
e) True

Radiology Review Manual. 5th edition. Dahnert. Lippincott, Williams and Wilkins, 2003: 787.

5 a) False - ulcerative colitis
b) False - few air fluid levels are seen. Plain abdominal radiograph appearances of a dilated transverse colon of greater than 5.5cm in diameter and pneumatosis coli
c) True
d) False - mortality of 20%
e) True

Radiology Review Manual. 5th edition. Dahnert. Lippincott, Williams and Wilkins, 2003: 861-2.

6 a) False - increased risk associated with Crohn's disease, coeliac disease, AIDS, systemic lupus erythematosus
b) True
c) False - diffuse involvement in 50%
d) False - caecum is most commonly involved
e) True

Radiology Review Manual. 5th edition. Dahnert. Lippincott, Williams and Wilkins, 2003: 841-2.

7 a) False - gastric acid levels are usually increased. Gastric ulcers are associated with a normal or low level of gastric acid
b) False - ulcers are bulbar in 95% and postbulbar in 3-5%. 50% are located in the anterior wall
c) False - less than 1mm in size. Giant duodenal ulcers >2cm are rare and have a higher risk of morbidity/mortality
d) False - perforation is a complication in <10%
e) True

Radiology Review Manual. 5th edition. Dahnert. Lippincott, Williams and Wilkins, 2003: 814.

8 a) False - found in the ileum 30%, oesophagus 20%, colon 15-30%, stomach 10%
b) False - right
c) True - there is an association with vertebral anomalies - spina bifida, hemivertebra and fusion defects
d) False - 60% occur in the distal oesophagus, 27% upper and 17% mid
e) True - posterior mediastinal mass +/- air fluid level

Radiology Review Manual. 5th edition. Dahnert. Lippincott, Williams and Wilkins, 2003: 816.

9 a) False
b) False
c) True
d) True - gaping ileocaecal valve in ulcerative colitis
e) False - deep ulcers commoner in Crohn's disease

Radiology Review Manual. 5th edition. Dahnert. Lippincott, Williams and Wilkins, 2003.

10 a) True
b) True
c) False
d) False
e) False

A Guide to Radiological Procedures. 4th edition. Chapman and Nakielny. W.B. Saunders, 2001: 53-5.

11 a) False
b) False
c) True
d) True
e) False

Radiology Review Manual. 5th edition. Dahnert. Lippincott, Williams and Wilkins, 2003: 829.

12 a) True - via the epiploic foramen
b) True
c) True
d) False - phrenicolic ligament attaches the descending colon to the left hemidiaphragm
e) False - greater curve

Radiology Review Manual. 5th edition. Dahnert. Lippincott, Williams and Wilkins, 2003: 784-6.

13 a) False - same preparation as barium enema
b) True
c) False - small faecal residue can be adherent to the wall. Small foci of faecal residue may also not contain gas bubbles, unlike larger foci
d) True
e) True

Taylor, *et al.* CT Colonography: Methods, Pathology and Pitfalls. *Clinical Radiology* 2003; 58 (3): 179-90.

14 a) True
b) True
c) True
d) True
e) True

Wong, *et al.* Helical CT Imaging of Clinically Suspected Appendicitis: Correlation of CT and Histological Findings. *Clinical Radiology* 2002; 57 (8): 741-5.

15 a) True
b) False - stomach
c) False
d) True
e) False - heterogenous with significant haemorrhage and necrosis

Kim, *et al.* Small Gastrointestinal Stromal Tumours with Focal Areas of Low Attenuation on CT: Pathological Correlation. *Clinical Radiology* 2005; 60 (3): 384-8.

16 a) True
b) False - squamous cell carcinoma
c) False - not seen
d) False - tumours below the dentate line spread to the inguinal lymph nodes. Tumours arising above, spread to perirectal and retroperitoneal nodes
e) True - reduced signal intensity on T1

Roach, *et al.* Magnetic Resonance Imaging of Anal Cancer. *Clinical Radiology* 2005; 60 (10): 1111-9.

17 a) False - 50-60%
b) False - left are commoner than right. Paraduodenal hernias are the commonest internal hernias. Small bowel herniates into Landzert's fossa to the left of the duodenum, which arises due to a defect in the descending mesocolon
c) False - proximal jejunum or duodenum
d) True
e) True

Sinha, Verma. Multidetector Row Computed Tomography in Bowel Obstruction. Part 1. Small Bowel Obstruction. *Clinical Radiology* 2005; 60 (10): 1058-67.

18 a) False - least commonly occurs in renal transplant patients. Commonest in heart-lung recipients
b) False - 1%
c) True
d) False - considerably more common
e) False - liver

Scarsbrook, *et al.* Post-Transplantation Lymphoproliferative Disorder: the Spectrum of Imaging Appearances. *Clinical Radiology* 2005; 60 (1): 47-55.

19 a) False
b) True
c) True
d) True - appendicitis is the other cause
e) False

Pereira, *et al.* Disproportionate Fat Stranding: a Helpful CT Sign in Patients with Acute Abdominal Pain. *RadioGraphics* 2004; 24: 703-5.

20 a) True - dilatation of oesophageal webs gives highest success rate
b) False - relieves dysphagia in 90%
c) True
d) True
e) False - migration occurs in up to 35%. Stents are more likely to migrate distally and most commonly occurs when the gastro-oeophageal junction is crossed

Therasse, *et al.* Balloon Dilatation and Stent Placement for Oesophageal Lesions. *RadioGraphics* 2003; 23: 89-105.

21 a) True
b) False - right lobe
c) False - indistinguishable on all pulse sequences
d) False - hypervascular. There is a significant risk of bleeding at biopsy
e) False - increases in size during pregnancy

Grazioli, *et al.* Hepatic Adenomas: Imaging and Pathologic Findings. *RadioGraphics* 2001; 21: 877.

22 a) True
b) True
c) True
d) True
e) False

Aids to Radiological Differential Diagnosis. 4th edition. Chapman and Nakielny. W.B. Saunders, 2003: 292-3.

23 a) False - occurs when part of the ventral bud fails to atrophy
b) True - other associations are tracheo-oesophageal fistula, oesophageal and duodenal atresia, and Down's syndrome
c) False - 85% involve the 2nd part of the duodenum, 15% involve 1st and 3rd
d) True
e) True - increased risk of peri-ampullary ulcers

Radiology Review Manual. 5th edition. Dahnert. Lippincott, Williams and Wilkins, 2003: 681-2.

24 a) False - intra and extrahepatic bile ducts are involved
b) False - almost always involved
c) True
d) True
e) False - feature of primary biliary cirrhosis

Radiology Review Manual. 5th edition. Dahnert. Lippincott, Williams and Wilkins, 2003: 697-8.

25 a) False - no recognised underlying risk factors
b) False - commonly 5-35-year-olds
c) False - central stellate calcification in 30-40%
d) False - reduced signal intensity on T1 and T2 weighted MRI images. In focal nodular hyperplasia there is reduced signal intensity on T1 and increased on T2
e) False - 90% mortality. Average survival of 6 months

Ichikawa, *et al.* Fibrolamellar Hepatocellular Carcinoma: Imaging and Pathologic Findings in 31 Recent Cases. *Radiology* 1999; 213: 352.

26 a) True
b) False - normal extrahepatic ducts
c) True
d) False - normal gallbladder
e) True

Blachar, *et al.* Primary Biliary Cirrhosis: Clinical, Pathologic, and Helical CT Findings in 53 Patients. *Radiology* 2001; 220: 329.

27 a) True - other liver features: cirrhosis, fatty infiltration, portal hypertension
b) False - hypoplastic gallbladder
c) True - other pancreatic features: calcifications, pancreatic cysts
d) False - microcolon with hyperplastic colonic mucosa
e) True

Radiology Review Manual. 5th edition. Dahnert. Lippincott, Williams and Wilkins, 2003: 481-2.

28 a) False - 15-30 minutes
b) True - 10% uptake by spleen, 5% bone marrow
c) True - reduced activity in the rest of the liver, so it is a relative hot spot
d) True - colloid shift seen in cirrhosis, hepatitis, chronic passive congestion and haematopoietic disorders
e) False - hot

Radiology Review Manual. 5th edition. Dahnert. Lippincott, Williams and Wilkins, 2003: 1109.

29 a) False - less than 5cm in size in 90%
b) False - hyperechoic, well defined lesions on ultrasound
c) True - reduced signal intensity on T1 weighted and increased on T2 weighted MR images
d) False - normal-sized arteries feeding with no AV shunting/ neovascularity
e) False - nodular peripheral enhancement early with complete filling in over 30 minutes

Fundamentals of Diagnostic Radiology. 2nd edition. Brant and Helms. Lippincott, Williams and Wilkins, 1999: 677.

30 a) True
b) True - can be an intraluminal soft tissue mass or focal/diffuse gallbladder wall thickening
c) False - 60% are located in the fundus
d) False - direct extension to the liver is the commonest mode of spread
e) False - 80% are adenocarcinomas

Fundamentals of Diagnostic Radiology. 2nd edition. Brant and Helms. Lippincott, Williams and Wilkins, 1999; Chapter 27: 687.
Radiology Review Manual. 5th edition. Dahnert. Lippincott, Williams and Wilkins, 2003: 705.

31 a) False - L1
b) True
c) False - <3-4mm
d) False - branch of the gastroduodenal artery from coeliac axis
e) False - 2mm proximal to the main duct

Anatomy for Diagnostic Imaging. 2nd edition. Ryan, McNichols and Eustace. W.B. Saunders, 2004: 181-3.

32
a) True - other contraindications: biliary tract sepsis and bleeding tendency
b) True
c) False - patient preparation with nil by mouth 5 hours prior to procedure, prophylactic antibiotics and check prothrombin time/platelets
d) False - mid-axillary
e) False - may be attempted up to 10 times

A Guide to Radiological Procedures. 4th edition. Chapman and Nakielny. W.B. Saunders, 2001: 116-8.

33
a) True
b) True
c) True
d) False - less than 4mm is normal. Common bile duct should measure 6mm or less in an adult
e) True

A Guide to Radiological Procedures. 4th edition. Chapman and Nakielny. W.B. Saunders, 2001: 124-6.

34
a) True
b) True
c) True
d) True
e) True

Radiology Review Manual. 5th edition. Dahnert. Lippincott, Williams and Wilkins, 2003: 726.

35
a) False - very rare
b) False - this is associated with liver angiosarcoma
c) True
d) False - 50-60 years
e) True

Thompson, *et al.* Angiosarcoma of the Spleen: Imaging Characteristics in 12 Patients. *Radiology* 2005; 235: 106-15.

36 a) True
b) True
c) False - can be normal in 30%
d) False - 24-48 hours
e) False - rare

Radiology Review Manual. 5th edition. Dahnert. Lippincott, Williams and Wilkins, 2003: 691.

37 a) False - this is normal. Abnormal <60cm/s
b) True
c) False - loss of pulsatility of portal flow is a sign of TIPS failure
d) True
e) True

Radiology Review Manual. 5th edition. Dahnert. Lippincott, Williams and Wilkins, 2003: 736.

38 a) True - hypertrophy of caudate lobe and segments 2 and 3. Shrinkage of right lobe and segments 4a and 4b
b) True - due to fatty infiltration
c) True - Doppler images resemble portal vein flow
d) True - with hyperintense septa
e) False - dilatation of the hepatic arteries

Radiology Review Manual. 5th edition. Dahnert. Lippincott, Williams and Wilkins, 2003: 696-7.

39 a) True
b) False - left gastric artery which is a branch of the coeliac axis. The inferior thyroid artery supplies the upper third and branches from the descending aorta supplies the middle third
c) False - posterior
d) True
e) True

Anatomy for Diagnostic Imaging. 2nd edition. Ryan, McNichols and Eustace. W.B. Saunders, 2004: 137-9.

40 a) True
b) False
c) True
d) True
e) True - other causes are ischaemic colitis, shistosomiasis, metastases to colon

Aids to Radiological Differential Diagnosis. 4th edition. Chapman and Nakielny. W.B. Saunders, 2003: 262.

Paper 4
Genitourinary, Adrenal, Obstetrics & Gynaecology and Breast

1 Concerning developmental abnormalities of the kidneys:

a) Duplication of the collecting system is seen in 10-12% of people
b) Accessory renal arteries normally enter the upper and mid poles
c) Horseshoe kidney is seen in 1 in 200 births
d) Horseshoe kidneys are more prone to trauma
e) Accessory renal arteries are less common in patients with horseshoe kidney

2 Glucagon is contraindicated in the following conditions:

a) Glucagonoma
b) Multiple myeloma
c) Sickle cell disease
d) Insulinoma
e) Phaeochromocytoma

3 The following are true of spiral (helical) CT scanning compared with sequential CT scanning:

a) There is reduction in partial volume artefacts
b) Reformatting into other planes is improved
c) The heat loading of the tube is lower
d) Noise is lower
e) There is less slice-to-slice misregistration

4 Causes of renal papillary necrosis include:

a) Aspirin
b) Diabetes mellitus
c) Sickle cell disease
d) Systemic lupus erythematosus
e) Sarcoidosis

5 The differential diagnosis of a pelvic fluid collection in a female on ultrasound includes:

a) Follicle rupture
b) Dermoid cyst
c) Ectopic pregnancy
d) Endometriosis
e) Pelvic inflammatory disease

6 Regarding ovarian cancer:

a) It is the commonest gynaecological malignancy
b) It is associated with colorectal cancer
c) CT only has a pre-operative staging accuracy of 50%
d) CA-125 is specific for ovarian cancer
e) Doppler ultrasound may help with differentiating benign from malignant disease

7 Regarding gestational trophoblastic disease:

a) Young maternal age is a risk factor
b) It is associated with theca-lutein cysts
c) A predominantly echo-poor mass is seen on ultrasound
d) Raised human chorionic gonadotrophin is seen in up to 80% of cases
e) Invasive mole develops in approximately half of cases

8 Causes of a thickened placenta on imaging include:

a) Diabetes
b) Infection
c) Rhesus incompatibility
d) Intra-uterine growth retardation
e) Gastroschisis

9 Regarding varicocoele embolisation:

a) The internal jugular vein may be punctured
b) The right spermatic vein joins the inferior vena cava just above the right renal vein
c) Should be limited to patients with large varicocoeles
d) Glyceryl-trinitrate may be needed
e) Embolisation is usually performed using polyvinyl alcohol particles

10 The following are true of ultrasound:

a) Resolution is improved by increasing frequency
b) M-mode imaging requires a high pulse rate frequency
c) In Doppler imaging the frequency of the approaching reflector decreases
d) Aliasing artefact is reduced by increasing frequency
e) Temperature rise of 1.5 degrees centigrade above normal produces no harmful effects regardless of duration

11 Angiomyolipoma:

a) Is a benign tumour
b) 50% are bilateral
c) CT demonstration of fat without calcification is diagnostic
d) Is characteristically hypoechoic on ultrasound
e) 20% of patients have tuberous sclerosis

12 The following cause bilateral large kidneys:

a) Acute glomerulonephritis
b) Amyloidosis
c) Uraemic medullary cystic disease
d) Diabetic glomerulosclerosis
e) Urate nephropathy

13 Regarding endometriosis:

a) Most commonly affects the fallopian tubes
b) 20% of infertile women are affected
c) Endometrioma is rarely anechoic on ultrasound
d) May present with pneumothorax
e) Cystic masses seen are typically hypointense on T1 weighted images

14 The following statements regarding breast disease are true:

a) Sclerosing adenosis is a risk factor for breast cancer
b) 10-15% of fibroadenomas undergo malignant change
c) A history of trauma is elicited in 80-85% of women presenting with fat necrosis of the breast
d) Gynaecomastia is bilateral in 15-20% of cases
e) Juvenile papillomatosis is associated with development of a metachronous tumour in 3-5%

15 The following are features of angiosarcoma of the breast:

a) Highly malignant breast tumour
b) Usually presents in women 50-60 years of age
c) Painful
d) Appears hyperechoic on ultrasound
e) Treatment requires mastectomy and axillary lymph node dissection

16 Features of cystosarcoma phylloides (phyllode tumour):

a) Slow growing mass
b) Commonly calcifies
c) Malignant degeneration occurs in 5-10%
d) Axillary metastases are rare
e) It usually presents in women under 20 years of age

17 Regarding breast cancer imaging:

a) 1-2% of breast cancers are mammographically occult
b) Germ line mutations are associated with an increased lifetime risk of developing breast cancer by 5-10%
c) BRCA 1 and 2 are the commonest germ line mutations associated with breast cancer
d) Breast cancer is most easily detected by mammography in women with dense breasts
e) Breast ultrasound uses a 10MHz high frequency probe

18 Regarding breast cancer metastases:

a) A long metastases-free interval is a good prognostic factor
b) Bony metastases have a better prognosis than lung metastases
c) Oestrogen receptor-positive metastases are more likely to occur in the liver
d) Peritoneal and retroperitoneal metastatic disease is more prevalent in lobular carcinomas of the breast
e) The site of initial metastastic deposits is more commonly the brain in those patients who have received adjuvant chemotherapy

19 Phaeochromocytoma:

a) When symptomatic tends to be larger at presentation
b) Is bilateral in 25%
c) Is associated with pulmonary hamartomas
d) Usually has CT attenuation values of <10 Hounsfield units (HU) on unenhanced scans
e) Is of high signal intensity on T2 weighted MR

20 Regarding benign and malignant adrenal masses:

a) Lesions >4cm tend to be malignant
b) Approximately one third of benign adenomas have HU of >10 on unenhanced CT
c) Adenomas tend to show delayed enhancement with IV contrast
d) Adenomas tend to show delayed clearance of IV contrast
e) Chemical shift MR utilises T1 weighted sequences

21 Concerning ovarian teratomas:

a) Mature teratomas are usually multi-loculated
b) Fat attenuation on CT is diagnostic for mature cystic teratoma
c) They are a known cause of peritonitis
d) Sebaceous fluid has low signal on T1 weighted MR
e) Calcification indicates a malignant teratoma

22 Regarding contrast media nephrotoxicity:

a) Old age is an independent risk factor
b) Development of nephrotoxicity is independent of dose given
c) Baseline creatinine must rise by 50% for the diagnosis to be made
d) Oral acetylcysteine is protective
e) Non-ionic dimmers are less nephrotoxic than low osmolar contrast media

23 Regarding ureteric stent placement:

a) Irritative bladder symptoms occur in over 75%
b) Encrustation is common when a stent is left for >6 weeks
c) Haematuria is a rare complication
d) Antibiotic prophylaxis is required even in the presence of a sterile urinary tract
e) Vesico-ureteric reflux is a common post-stent complication

24 Omphalocoele:

a) Is a midline abdominal wall defect
b) Has no covering over the herniated contents
c) Is usually an isolated abnormality
d) Is associated with a normal umbilical cord insertion
e) Is associated with Beckwith-Wiedemann syndrome

25 Regarding renal lymphoma:
a) Primary renal lymphoma is rare
b) It is more common in non-Hodgkin's lymphoma
c) It is hypoechoic at ultrasound
d) Multiple masses are more common than isolated lesions
e) Post-contrast, there is decreased enhancement compared to the surrounding normal renal parenchyma

26 Multicystic dysplastic kidney:
a) Is the second commonest cause of a neonatal abdominal mass
b) Is usually unilateral
c) Is associated with PUJ obstruction
d) The renal cysts communicate
e) Intervening normal renal parenchyma is present

27 Medial deviation of the ureters is caused by:
a) Iliopsoas hypertrophy
b) Retrocaval ureter
c) Aortic aneurysm
d) Retroperitoneal fibrosis
e) Pelvic lipomatosis

28 Regarding emphysematous infections of the renal tract:
a) Diabetes is present in almost half the cases of pyelonephritis
b) *Escherichia coli* is the most common pathogen
c) Infection does not spread beyond the renal capsule
d) Ultrasound reliably demonstrates the depth of involvement
e) Perirenal fluid collections are a poor prognostic sign

29 Regarding paratesticular masses:
a) Epididymal cysts are anechoic at ultrasound
b) Spermatocoeles may be distinguished from epididymal cysts by ultrasound
c) Papillary cystadenomas are associated with cerebellar haemangiomas
d) Pampiniform plexus vessel diameter of 4mm is normal
e) Lipomas are the most common paratesticular tumour

30 Regarding prostatic carcinoma:

a) Zonal anatomy is best depicted on T2 weighted MR
b) The prostatic capsule is of low signal intensity on T2 weighted MR
c) Carcinoma is usually intermediate to high signal on T2 weighted MR
d) Haemorrhage may mimic carcinoma
e) The vas deferens and seminal vesicles are of high T2 signal intensity

1 a) False - 4%
b) False - lower pole below the hilum
c) False - 1 in 700 births
d) True - as they lie across the vertebral column
e) False - more common

Anatomy for Diagnostic Imaging. 2nd edition. Ryan, McNichols and Eustace. W.B. Saunders, 2004: 189-92.

2 a) True
b) False
c) False
d) True
e) True

A Guide to Radiological Procedures. 4th edition. Chapman and Nakielny. W.B. Saunders, 2001: 63-9.

3 a) True
b) True
c) False - higher as there are no cooling periods between slices
d) False - higher
e) True

Physics for Medical Imaging. Farr, Allisy-Roberts. Bailliere Tindell, 1996: 114.

4 a) True
b) True - accounts for 50% of cases
c) True
d) False
e) False

Aids to Radiological Differential Diagnosis. 4th edition. Chapman and Nakielny. W.B. Saunders, 2003: 338-9.

5 a) True
b) True
c) True
d) True
e) True

Textbook of Radiology and Imaging. 7th edition. Sutton. Churchill Livingstone, 2002: 989-1017.

6 a) False - second commonest after endometrial carcinoma
b) True - Lynch Type 2 cancer family syndrome
c) False - 70-90%
d) False - elevated in benign conditions, e.g. fibroids, endometriosis and pelvic inflammatory disease
e) True

Radiology Review Manual. 5th edition. Dahnert. Lippincott, Williams and Wilkins, 2003: 1046-8.

7 a) False - increased maternal age
b) True - in 20-50% of patients
c) False - echogenic mass
d) False - 100%
e) False - 12-15% of cases

Aids to Radiological Differential Diagnosis. 4th edition. Chapman and Nakielny. W.B. Saunders, 2003: 514-5.

8 a) True
b) True
c) True
d) False
e) False

Aids to Radiological Differential Diagnosis. 4th edition. Chapman and Nakielny. W.B. Saunders, 2003: 513.

9 a) True - although the common femoral vein is often used
b) False - it joins the anterior aspect of the inferior vena cava just below the right renal vein
c) False - symptomatic or subfertile patients
d) True - if the spermatic vein goes into spasm
e) False - using coils

Interventional Radiology, a Survival Guide. 2nd edition. Kessel, Robertson. Elsevier, 2005: 204-5.

10 a) True
b) True - used in echocardiography
c) False - increases
d) False
e) True

Physics for Medical Imaging. Farr, Allisy-Roberts. Bailliere Tindell, 1996: 183-213.

11 a) True - however, patients may die from massive haemorrhage
b) False - 80% are unilateral
c) True
d) False - characteristically hyperechoic
e) True

Fundamentals of Diagnostic Radiology. 2nd edition. Brant and Helms. Lippincott, Williams and Wilkins, 1999: 779-80.

12 a) True
b) True
c) False - causes bilateral small kidneys
d) True
e) True

Fundamentals of Diagnostic Radiology. 2nd edition. Brant and Helms. Lippincott, Williams and Wilkins, 1999: 789.

13 a) False - 80% affects the ovaries
b) True
c) True - classically has diffuse low-level internal echoes
d) True
e) False - homogenously hyperintense on T1 weighted images

Radiology Review Manual. 5th edition. Dahnert. Lippincott, Williams and Wilkins, 2003: 1032-4.

14 a) False
b) False - this is a benign tumour
c) False - 40%
d) False - bilateral in 60-65%
e) True

Radiology Review Manual. 5th edition. Dahnert. Lippincott, Williams and Wilkins, 2003: 548-56.

15 a) True
b) False - women 20-30 years of age
c) False - painless
d) False - it is a well defined multilobulated hypoechoic mass. If there is haemorrhage then it can contain hyperechoic areas
e) False - haematogenous spread. There is no spread by lymphatics

Radiology Review Manual. 5th edition. Dahnert. Lippincott, Williams and Wilkins, 2003: 548-65.

16 a) False - rapidly enlarging mass
b) False
c) True
d) True
e) False - usually presents in 5th-6th decade

Radiology Review Manual. 5th edition. Dahnert. Lippincott, Williams and Wilkins, 2003: 548-57.

17 a) False - 10-12%
b) False - increased lifetime risk of developing breast cancer by 60-80%. More than 50% are afflicted before 50 years of age
c) True
d) False - less likely to be detected in women with dense breasts and <50 years of age
e) True

Sim, *et al.* US Correlation for MRI-detected Breast Lesions in Women with Familial Risk of Breast Cancer. *Clinical Radiology* 2005; 60 (7): 801-6.

18 a) True
b) True
c) False - more likely to occur in bone
d) True - as are gastrointestinal and gynaecological
e) True - since the majority of chemotherapy agents used in the treatment of breast cancer do not cross the blood-brain barrier

Porter, *et al.* Patterns of Metastatic Breast Carcinoma: Influence of Tumour Histological Grade. *Clinical Radiology* 2004; 59 (12): 1094-8.

19 a) False - symptomatic tumours tend to be smaller at presentation
b) False - 10% bilateral, 10% malignant
c) True - as part of the Carney triad
d) False - they rarely contain sufficient fat for HU to be <10
e) True

Blake, Kalra, *et al.* Phaeochromocytoma: An Imaging Chameleon. *RadioGraphics* 2004; 24: 587-99.

20 a) True
b) True
c) False - adenomas enhance rapidly
d) False - adenomas show rapid washout of contrast media
e) True

Mayo-Smith, Boland, *et al.* State of the Art Adrenal Imaging. *RadioGraphics* 2001; 21: 995-1012.

21 a) False - unilocular
b) True
c) True - following rupture or torsion
d) False - high T1 signal intensity
e) False - calcification outside the mural nodule is suspicious of malignancy

Jung, Lee, *et al.* CT and MRI of Ovarian Tumours with Emphasis on Differential Diagnosis. *RadioGraphics* 2002; 22: 1305-25.

22 a) True - as are diabetic nephropathy, dehydration, heart failure and NSAIDS
b) False - nephrotoxicity is dose-dependent
c) False - 25% above baseline levels
d) True
e) True

Morcos. Prevention of Contrast Media Nephrotoxicity - The Story So Far. *Clinical Radiology* 2004; 59: 381-9.

23 a) True
b) True - 47% at 6-12 weeks
c) False - microscopic haematuria is seen following most stents
d) True
e) True - 80% of cases

Dyer, Chen, *et al.* Complication of Ureteral Stent Placement. *RadioGraphics* 2002; 22: 1005-22.

24 a) True
b) False - covered by peritoneum and amnion
c) False - other anomalies in over 80% of cases
d) False
e) True

O`Connor, Levine. Beckwith-Wiedemann Syndrome. *Radiology* 2002; 224: 375-8.

25 a) True
b) True
c) True
d) True
e) True

Urban, Fishman. Renal Lymphoma: CT Patterns with Emphasis on Helical CT. *RadioGraphics* 2000; 20: 197-212.

26 a) True - hydronephrosis is the most common cause
b) True
c) True - in 10 - 20% of cases
d) False - no communication is seen
e) False - no normal renal parenchyma is seen

Mercado-Deane, Beeson. US of Renal Insufficiency in Neonates. *RadioGraphics* 2002; 22: 1429-38.

27 a) True
b) True - right side only
c) False - lateral deviation
d) True
e) True

Radiology Review Manual. 5th edition. Dahnert. Lippincott, Williams and Wilkins, 2003: 886.

28 a) False - in over 90%
b) True
c) False - gas may extend into the perirenal space
d) False - CT is more effective
e) False - perirenal fluid collections imply a favourable immune response

Grayson, Abbott, *et al.* Emphysematous Infections of the Abdomen and Pelvis: A Pictorial Review. *RadioGraphics* 2002; 22: 543-61.

29 a) True
b) False - both are well defined, anechoic structures
c) True - as part of von Hippel-Lindau disease
d) False - >3mm is abnormal
e) True

Woodward, Schwab, *et al.* Extratesticular Scrotal Masses: Radiologic - Pathologic Correlation. *RadioGraphics* 2003; 23: 215-40.

30 a) True
b) True
c) False - low signal intensity
d) True - as may prostatitis, hyperplastic nodules and radiation therapy
e) True

Claus, Hricak, *et al.* Pretreatment Evaluation of Prostate Cancer: Role of MR Imaging and MR Spectroscopy. *RadioGraphics* 2004; 24: S167-S180.

Paper 5

Paediatrics

1 Ewing's sarcoma:

a) Most commonly affects children and adolescents
b) Readily metastasises to bone
c) Is usually medullary in origin
d) Is of low signal on T1 weighted MRI
e) Is iso-intense to skeletal muscle on T2 weighted MRI

2 Down's sydrome is associated with:

a) Accelerated sutural closure
b) Atlanto-axial subluxation
c) Anterior vertebral body scalloping
d) Hirschprung's disease
e) Annular pancreas

3 On neonatal cranial ultrasound:

a) The cerebellar vermis is typically hypoechoic
b) Choroid plexus is highly echogenic
c) Ventricles are usually slit-like in the premature infant
d) Cavum septum pellucidum is rarely seen in the term infant
e) The caudothalamic groove is a rare place for intracranial haemorrhage

4 Clinical and radiological features of neurofibromatosis Type 1 include:

a) Unilateral limb overgrowth
b) Inferior rib notching
c) Pseudoarthroses of long bones
d) Coarctation of the aorta
e) Multiple meningiomas

5 Hypertrophic pyloric stenosis:

a) Hypertrophied pyloric muscle is hypoechoic on ultrasound
b) Pyloric muscle thickness >4mm is abnormal
c) Pyloric transverse diameter of 12mm is normal
d) Male infants are more frequently affected
e) The stomach is usually atonic

6 Regarding childhood liver tumours:

a) Hepatocellular carcinoma typically occurs over 5 years of age
b) Hepatoblastoma is more common <2 years of age
c) Hepatoblastoma is associated with hemihypertrophy
d) Hepatocellular carcinoma is a complication of biliary atresia
e) Hepatocellular carcinoma typically causes a cold spot on HIDA scanning

7 Concerning imaging of the testis:

a) An appendix testis is present in over 90% of males
b) Examination of the contralateral testis is mandatory in possible torsion
c) A hydrocoele may cause false positive diagnosis of torsion on scintigraphic evaluation
d) A torted testis is usually of high echogenicity on ultrasound
e) Torsion is most common in the neonatal age group

8 Regarding imaging of the adrenal glands:

a) At birth, the adrenal glands are around one third the size of the adjacent kidney
b) The limb of a mature adrenal gland should not measure more than 5mm
c) In renal agenesis, the adrenal gland assumes a discoid shape
d) Childhood adrenocortical neoplasms are hyperintense on T2 weighted MRI
e) Ectopic adrenal tissue is typically sited around the superior mesenteric artery

9 Concerning imaging of the complications of renal transplantation:

a) Acute rejection occurs in up to 40% of cases
b) Ultrasound reliably differentiates acute rejection from tubular necrosis
c) On colour Doppler imaging, a resistive index of >0.9 is abnormal
d) Arterial thrombosis is more common than venous
e) Obstruction in the early postoperative period is usually due to the ureteric anastomosis

10 Regarding solid abdominal malignancy in childhood:

a) Wilms' tumours are bilateral in up to 25%
b) Neuroblastomas are associated with hemihypertrophy
c) Neuroblastomas calcify in over 80% on CT
d) Wilms' tumours tend to encase the central vascular structures
e) Wilms' tumours are more common in horseshoe kidneys

11 The following are features of osteogenesis imperfecta:

a) Most cases involve an autosomal dominant mode of inheritance
b) Multiple wormian bones
c) Dense, sclerotic bones
d) Exuberant callus formation around fractures
e) Basilar invagination

12 Regarding developmental dysplasia of the hip:

a) The condition is more common in breech presentation
b) It is usually bilateral
c) Ultrasound is performed in the coronal plane
d) The acetabular labrum is hypoechoic on ultrasound
e) Hilgenreiners line should pass through both triradiate cartilages on plain films

13 Radiological features of rickets include:

a) Radiological signs indicate the underlying aetiology
b) Widening of the growth plate as a late sign
c) Bulbous anterior rib ends
d) A sclerotic rim surrounding the epiphysis
e) Dense metaphyseal bands

14 In craniosynostosis:

a) The skull vault is formed by membranous ossification
b) Single sutural synostosis is more common than multiple
c) Overall, 15% of cases are syndromic in nature
d) Sagittal synostosis results in a trigonocephalic skull
e) Bilateral coronal synostosis results in a brachycephalic skull

15 Radiological features of absent corpus callosum include:

a) Crescentic lateral ventricles
b) A high riding third ventricle
c) Enlargement of the occipital horns
d) Hypoplasia of the optic nerves
e) Separation of pericallosal arteries on angiography

16 Concerning abnormalities of intestinal rotation:

a) The midgut extends from the duodenojejunal flexure to the ascending colon
b) During development, the midgut rotates 270 degress clockwise around the superior mesenteric artery axis
c) Ladd's bands are a cause of low intestinal obstruction
d) The duodenojejunal flexure should lie at the level of the pylorus on barium studies
e) The superior mesenteric vein normally lies to the left of the artery

17 The normal thymus:

a) Develops from the third branchial pouch
b) May enlarge following illness
c) CT density (Hounsfield units) increases with increasing age
d) On T1 weighted MRI the gland is iso-intense to mediastinal fat
e) Reaches a maximum size in the 2nd decade

18 Regarding MRI signal characteristics:

a) T1 signal is produced by longtitudinal relaxation
b) Cerebral grey matter has intermediate T1 signal intensity
c) Cerebrospinal fluid has a long T2 relaxation time
d) Spin echo sequences begin with a 180 degree radiofrequency pulse
e) Inversion recovery sequences begin with an initial 90 degree radiofrequency pulse

19 Radiological findings in tetralogy of Fallot typically include:

a) A large ASD
b) Overriding of the aorta
c) Right ventricular hypoplasia
d) Pulmonary plethora
e) Aortic valve stenosis

20 Radiological findings in sickle cell disease include:

a) 'Hair-on-end' skull appearance
b) Premature conversion of red to fatty bone marrow
c) Subperiosteal new bone formation in the tubular bones of the hand and feet
d) Salmonella osteomyelitis
e) Enlarged kidneys

21 Portal venous gas may be seen in which of the following conditions:

a) Pneumonia
b) Imperforate anus
c) Duodenal atresia
d) Necrotising enterocolitis
e) Umbilical catheterisation

22 Air trapping may be seen in:

a) Asthma
b) Bronchogenic cyst
c) Intalobar sequestration
d) Langerhans' cell histiocytosis
e) Inhaled foreign body

23 Features of Swyer-James syndrome include:

a) Increased lucency of a hemithorax
b) Increased hilar markings, with peripheral pruning
c) Air trapping during expiration
d) Mild bronchiectasis
e) Typically a lobar or segmental distribution

24 Regarding a double aortic arch:

a) It is the most common vascular ring
b) The descending aorta is usually on the left side
c) The left aortic arch is usually higher than the right
d) The left aortic arch is usually larger than the right
e) It is often associated with other congenital anomalies

25 Regarding paediatric ependymomas:

a) Tumours usually arise from the cerebellar hemispheres
b) Tumours are more frequently supratentorial
c) Tumours commonly extend through the foramen of Magendie
d) MR signal is characteristic
e) Calcification is seen in up to 50%

26 Concerning infrahepatic interruption of the inferior vena cava:

a) It involves absence of the IVC between the renal vessels and right atrium
b) Venous drainage is predominantly via the left azygous system
c) The hepatic veins drain into the left atrium
d) There is an association with anomalous pulmonary venous drainage
e) There is an association with polysplenia

27 Dysembryoplastic neuroepithelial tumours:

a) Rarely present with seizures
b) Typically arise in the periventricular region
c) Usually arise in the parieto-occipital region
d) Are hypodense on unenhanced CT
e) Produce extensive surrounding oedema

28 Regarding the Dandy-Walker malformation:

a) The posterior fossa is small
b) There is a high lying tentorium
c) The cerebellar vermis is normal
d) The corpus callosum is absent in up to 25%
e) There is inferior displacement of the vein of Galen

29 The following cause anterior oesophageal impression on barium swallow:

a) Aberrant left subclavian vein
b) Aberrant left pulmonary artery
c) Double aortic arch
d) Left atrial enlargement
e) Right aortic arch with mirror image branching

30 Regarding congenital cystic adenomatoid malformation:
a) The abnormality is purely cystic in nature
b) Cysts usually communicate with the bronchial tree
c) Mediastinal shift is toward the affected lung
d) Abdominal radiographs reveal a scaphoid abdomen
e) It is associated with pulmonary sequestration

1 a) True - 75% are <20 years of age, with most being 5-15
b) True
c) True - mostly diaphyseal in origin (25% metaphyseal)
d) True - allows the extent of marrow involvement to be assessed
e) False - hyperintense to skeletal muscle on T2 sequences

Diagnostic Radiology. A Textbook of Medical Imaging. 4th edition. Grainger and Allison. Churchill Livingstone, 2001: 1890-2.

2 a) False - delayed sutural closure, with a persistent metopic suture in 40-79%
b) True
c) True
d) True
e) True

Radiology Review Manual. 5th edition. Dahnert. Lippincott, Williams and Wilkins, 2003: 68.

3 a) False - the cerebellum is usually hypoechoic
b) True
c) False - ventricles are prominent in premature infants
d) False - seen in over 50% of term neonates
e) False - a common location for intracerebral haemorrhage

Pediatric Neuroimaging. 4th edition. AJ Barkovich. Lippincott Williams & Wilkins, 2005.

4 a) True
b) True
c) True
d) True
e) False - a feature of neurofibromatosis Type 2

Diagnostic Radiology. A Textbook of Medical Imaging. 4th edition. Grainger and Allison. Churchill Livingstone, 2001: 2347-9.

5 a) True
b) True
c) True
d) True
e) False - exaggerated peristaltic waves

Radiology Review Manual. 5th edition. Dahnert. Lippincott, Williams and Wilkins, 2003: 832-4.

6 a) True - peak age 12-14 years of age
b) True
c) True
d) True
e) False - hot spots, although atypical / cold spots may be seen

Radiology Review Manual. 5th edition. Dahnert. Lippincott, Williams and Wilkins, 2003: 713-5.

7 a) True
b) True
c) True
d) False - hypoechoic due to congestion, infarction and oedema
e) False - rare in neonates

Sidhu. Clinical and Imaging Features of Testicular Torsion: The Role of Ultrasound. *Clinical Radiology* 1999; 54: 343-52.

8 a) True
b) True
c) True
d) True
e) False - around the adrenal bed, or the coeliac axis

Barwick, Mulhotra, *et al.* Embryology of the Adrenal Glands and Relevance to Diagnostic Imaging. *Clinical Radiology* 2005; 60: 953-9.

9 a) True
b) False
c) True - this may occur in both acute tubular necrosis or acute rejection
d) False - arterial thrombosis is rare
e) False - obstruction within 72 hours is usually due to blood clots

Baxter. Ultrasound of Renal Transplantation. *Clinical Radiology* 2001; 56: 802-18.

10 a) False - bilateral in up to 10%
b) False - Wilms' tumours are associated with hemihypertrophy
c) True
d) False - displace
e) True - also with aniridia, hemihypertrophy and cryptorchidism

Radiology Review Manual. 5th edition. Dahnert. Lippincott, Williams and Wilkins, 2003: 984.

11 a) True
b) True
c) False - diffuse demineralisation and cortical thinning
d) True
e) True

Textbook of Radiology and Imaging. 7th edition. Sutton. Churchill Livingstone, 2002: 1124-6.

12 a) True
b) False - unilateral is 11 times more common
c) True
d) False - acetabular labrum is echogenic. Femoral head is hypoechoic
e) True

Radiology Review Manual. 5th edition. Dahnert. Lippincott, Williams and Wilkins, 2003.

13 a) False - radiological features are similar regardless of underlying cause
b) False - an early sign
c) True - the 'richetic rosary' sign
d) False - this is seen in scurvy
e) True

Textbook of Radiology and Imaging. 7th edition. Sutton. Churchill Livingstone, 2002: 1352-4.

14 a) True - enchondral ossification occurs in the skull base
b) True - 60% of cases
c) True
d) False - scaphocephalic skull
e) True

Pediatric Neuroimaging. 4th edition. AJ Barkovich. Lippincott Williams & Wilkins, 2005: 410-20.

15 a) True
b) True
c) True
d) True
e) True

Radiology Review Manual. 5th edition. Dahnert. Lippincott, Williams and Wilkins, 2003: 258-9.

16 a) False - duodenojejunal flexure to mid-transverse colon
b) False - anti-clockwise
c) False - high intestinal obstruction
d) True
e) False - superior mesenteric vein should lie to the right of the superior mesenteric artery

Diagnostic Radiology. A Textbook of Medical Imaging. 4th edition. Grainger and Allison. Churchill Livingstone, 2001: 1149-51.

17 a) True
b) True
c) False - decreases with age (fatty replacement)
d) False - hypointense to surrounding fat on T1 sequences
e) True

Aids to Radiological Differential Diagnosis. 4th edition. Chapman and Nakielny. W.B. Saunders, 2003: 178-9.

18 a) False - T1 signal is produced by transverse relaxation
b) True
c) True
d) False - 90 degree pulse, with multiple subsequent 180 degree pulses
e) False - an initial 180 degree pulse

Pooles. Fundamental Physics of MR Imaging. *RadioGraphics* 2005 24(4): 1087-99.

19 a) False - a large (subvalvular) VSD is typical
b) True
c) False - right ventricular hypertrophy
d) False - pulmonary oligaemia
e) False - pulmonary stenosis

Mirowitz, *et al.* Tetralogy of Fallot: MR Findings. *Radiology* 1989; 171: 207.

20 a) True
b) False - delayed conversion of red to fatty bone marrow
c) True - often the earliest radiological manifestation
d) True
e) True - due to increased perfusion secondary to anaemia. Also, reduced size in late disease due to infarcts

Lonergan, *et al.* Sickle Cell Anaemia. *RadioGraphics* 2001; 21: 971-94.

21 a) True
b) True
c) True
d) True
e) True

Radiology Review Manual. 5th edition. Dahnert. Lippincott, Williams and Wilkins, 2003: 661.

22 a) True
b) True
c) False
d) True
e) True

Diagnostic Radiology. A Textbook of Medical Imaging. 4th edition. Grainger and Allison. Churchill Livingstone, 2001.

23 a) True
b) False
c) True
d) True
e) False - usually the entire lung is affected

Diagnostic Radiology. A Textbook of Medical Imaging. 4th edition. Grainger and Allison. Churchill Livingstone, 2001: 652.

24 a) True
b) True - in 75%
c) False - the right arch normally lies higher than the left arch
d) False - the right arch is normally larger
e) False - it is usually an isolated anomaly

Radiology Review Manual. 5th edition. Dahnert. Lippincott, Williams and Wilkins, 2003: 577.

25 a) False - the 4th ventricle
b) False - infratentorial in 70%
c) True
d) False
e) True

Pediatric Neuroimaging. 4th edition. AJ Barkovich. Lippincott Williams & Wilkins, 2005: 525-7.

26 a) True
b) False - the right azygous vein
c) False - the right atrium
d) True
e) True

Diagnostic Radiology. A Textbook of Medical Imaging. 4th edition. Grainger and Allison. Churchill Livingstone, 2001: 821.

27 a) False - presentation is usually with refractory seizures
b) False - cortical and subcortical grey matter
c) True
d) False - temporal lobe in 60%, frontal in 30%
e) False - surrounding oedema is atypical

Radiology Review Manual. 5th edition. Dahnert. Lippincott, Williams and Wilkins, 2003: 276-7.

28 a) False - the posterior fossa is enlarged
b) True
c) False - hypoplastic or absent vermis
d) True
e) False - superior displacement of the vein of Galen

Diagnostic Radiology. A Textbook of Medical Imaging. 4th edition. Grainger and Allison. Churchill Livingstone, 2001: 2487-8.

29 a) False - posterior impression
b) True
c) True
d) True
e) False - normal barium swallow

Radiology Review Manual. 5th edition. Dahnert. Lippincott, Williams and Wilkins, 2003: 577-80.

30 a) False - solid and cystic elements
b) True
c) False - typically away from the affected side
d) False - a feature of congenital diaphragmatic hernias
e) True

Diagnostic Radiology. A Textbook of Medical Imaging. 4th edition. Grainger and Allison. Churchill Livingstone, 2001: 639-40, 654.

Paper 6
Central Nervous System and Head & Neck

1 Regarding sonography of normal neck lymph nodes:

a) There are a total of 100 lymph nodes in the neck
b) At least 5 or 6 normal cervical nodes are identified routinely by sonography of the neck
c) The number of normal cervical lymph nodes that can be detected by ultrasound decreases with advancing age
d) There is an increase in intranodal fatty infiltration with age
e) The normal submandibular and parotid nodes are usually round

2 The following are branches of the vertebral artery:

a) Anterior spinal artery
b) Anterior inferior cerebellar artery
c) Posterior inferior cerebellar artery
d) Superior cerebellar artery
e) Pontine artery

3 Concerning the differentiation between optic nerve glioma and optic nerve sheath meningioma:

a) Optic nerve sheath meningioma affects an older age group
b) A widened optic canal is seen more commonly in optic nerve glioma
c) Calcification is more commonly seen with optic nerve glioma
d) Optic nerve glioma typically shows the 'tram-track' sign on enhancement
e) Optic nerve glioma may cause orbital hyperostosis

4 Regarding the parathyroid glands:

a) Fewer than 2% of superior parathyroid glands are ectopic in location
b) The reported sensitivity of ultrasound in detection of parathyroid adenoma is only 40-45%
c) The parathyroid glands arise from the 3rd and 4th branchial pouches
d) Spin-echo T2 weighted MRI in the coronal plane is the most sensitive imaging sequence for detection of parathyroid adenoma
e) Typically, parathyroid adenoma is seen as a homogenous hyperechoic nodule on ultrasound

5 The basal ganglia consist of the following:

a) Corpus striatum
b) Claustrum
c) Fornix
d) Hippocampus
e) Amygdaloid body

6 Concerning intracranial lymphoma:

a) It is usually a Hodgkin's lymphoma
b) Secondary lymphoma more commonly involves the leptomeninges than the brain parenchyma
c) It is usually hypodense on unenhanced CT
d) It is normally high signal on T2 weighted images
e) Toxoplasmosis may mimic lymphoma in the brain

7 Causes of loss of the lamina dura of the teeth include:

a) Osteomalacia
b) Hyperparathyroidism
c) Scleroderma
d) Langerhans' cell histiocytosis
e) Paget's disease

8 Regarding fibro-osseous lesions of the face and jaw:

a) Periosteal reaction is not a feature of benign fibro-osseous lesions
b) The monostatic form accounts for 40-50% of cases of fibrous dysplasia
c) In fibrous dysplasia the teeth generally remain undisplaced with resorption
d) Most cemento-ossifying fibromas are treated surgically
e) Site predilection of fibrous dysplasia is for the mandible

9 Concerning glial tumours of the brain:

a) They account for 40-45% of all intracranial tumours
b) Low grade astrocytomas usually enhance
c) Glioblastoma multiforme is the most common and most malignant glioma
d) Calcification is seen in up to 40% of oligodendrogliomas on CT
e) Oligodendroglioma most commonly affects the parietal and occipital lobes

10 Concerning posterior fossa tumours in children:

a) 80% of medulloblastomas arise from the vermis
b) Juvenile pilocytic astrocytomas are the second commonest posterior fossa tumour
c) Juvenile pilocytic astrocytomas usually calcify
d) Brainstem gliomas mostly affect the midbrain
e) Ependymoma seeds to the CSF in 30% of cases

11 The following are true regarding multiple sclerosis:

a) Periventricular lesions are aligned parallel to the long axis of the lateral ventricles
b) The thoracic cord is the most common part of the spinal cord to be affected
c) Lesions are typically bright on T2 weighted MRI
d) 40% of spinal cord lesions have associated brain lesions
e) Most spinal cord lesions are low signal on T1 weighted MRI

12 Concerning intraorbital pathology:

a) Optic nerve glioma is the commonest tumour arising from the optic nerve sheath complex
b) Idiopathic inflammatory pseudotumour is unilateral in 40-50% of cases in adults
c) The lacrimal gland is the most frequently involved orbital structure in idiopathic inflammatory pseudotumour
d) Use of steroids differentiates idiopathic inflammatory pseudotumour from lymphoma
e) Thyroid eye disease is the most common disorder affecting the orbit

13 Regarding paragangliomas:

a) They can arise anywhere from the base of skull to the floor of the pelvis
b) They usually enhance intensely with contrast
c) Glomus jugulare tumours typically produce a 'salt and pepper' appearance on CT
d) Glomus tympanicum tumour is the commonest tumour in the middle ear
e) Glomus vagale tumour most commonly affects the vagus nerve within the base of the skull at the level of the jugular bulb

14 The following are causes of white matter demyelination:

a) Behcet's disease
b) Moya-moya disease
c) Lyme disease
d) Marchiafava-bignami syndrome
e) Subacute sclerosing panencephalitis

15 The following are correct concerning MRI:

a) Spin-echo sequences use 180 degree pulses
b) Gradient-echo sequences use 180 degree pulses
c) Gradient-echo sequences have lower noise compared with spin-echo
d) Echo planar imaging is a fast spin-echo sequence
e) Spatial resolution of MRI is 2 line pairs per mm

16 The following are true regarding meningitis:
a) *Neisseria meningitides* is the commonest cause in children
b) Subdural effusions are common in infants with *Haemophilus influenzae*
c) Leptomeningeal enhancement is more marked in tuberculosis than bacterial meningitis
d) Hydrocephalus is commonly seen in fungal meningitis
e) Group B haemolytic streptococcus is the commonest cause in neonates

17 The following are branches of the external carotid artery:
a) Ascending pharyngeal artery
b) Inferior thyroid artery
c) Posterior auricular artery
d) Occipital artery
e) Lingual artery

18 Concerning neurodegenerative disorders:
a) Marked enlargement of the temporal horns is seen in Alzheimer's disease
b) Thinning of the pars reticularis is seen on MRI in Parkinsonism
c) Huntington's disease is inherited in autosomal dominant fashion
d) In Huntington's disease, atrophy most severely affects the caudate nucleus
e) The Kayser-Fleischer ring is virtually diagnostic of Huntington's disease

19 Choroid plexus papilloma:
a) Causes increased production of cerebrospinal fluid
b) Is usually hypodense on unenhanced CT
c) Usually affects the 4th ventricle in adults
d) Is usually low signal on T2 weighted MRI
e) Undergoes malignant degeneration in 2-4%

20 The following will increase signal-to-noise ratio in MRI:

a) Decreasing the matrix size
b) More signal averages
c) Wide receiver bandwidth
d) Increased repetition time
e) Decreasing field strength

21 Juvenile angiofibroma:

a) Is the commonest benign nasopharyngeal tumour
b) Almost exclusively affects females
c) Widening of the pterygopalatine fossa is only seen in advanced cases
d) Biopsy is contraindicated
e) Invasion of the sphenoid sinus occurs in up to two thirds of cases

22 Concerning normal anatomy of the temporal bone:

a) The lateral two thirds of the external auditory canal are cartilaginous
b) The epitympanum contains the malleo-incudal articulation
c) The roof of the epitympanum forms the sinus tympani
d) The tympanic portion of the facial nerve runs posterolaterally and inferior to the lateral semicircular canal
e) The stapes footplate sits in the round window nidus

23 Concerning neurilemmoma (acoustic neuroma):

a) It is the third commonest neoplasm of the cerebellopontine angle
b) The sporadic form is more common in females
c) Bilateral tumours allow a presumptive diagnosis of Type 2 neurofibromatosis
d) It arises from the vestibular portion of the nerve in 85%
e) It is hypointense on T2 weighted MRI

24 Regarding sonography of abnormal neck lymph nodes:

a) Regardless of the primary tumour, the presence of a metastatic node reduces the 5-year survival rate by 50%
b) Malignant nodes have sharp borders, whereas benign nodes usually have unsharp borders
c) Metastatic nodes are usually hyperechoic when compared to the adjacent muscles
d) Nodal calcification is common in metastatic nodes from follicular carcinoma of the thyroid
e) The presence of peripheral vascularity is highly suggestive of malignancy

25 The following are true concerning variants of the circle of Willis:

a) A 'foetal' posterior communicating artery is seen in up to 60-70% of people
b) The anterior cerebral artery may be fused as a single trunk
c) A hypoplastic anterior communicating artery is seen in 20% of people
d) Variation of at least one vessel, enough to affect its role as a collateral route, is found in 60% of people
e) The circle of Willis is complete in 90% of people

26 Regarding viral central nervous system infections:

a) CSF aspirate is usually negative in *Herpes simplex* encephalitis
b) Decreased density of the temporal lobe on CT with sparing of the putamen is typical of *Herpes simplex* encephalitis
c) Creutzfeldt-Jakob disease causes areas of high signal in the basal ganglia on T2 weighted MRI
d) In *Varicella zoster*, cerebral infarcts are seen on the same side as the skin manifestations
e) Acute disseminated encephalomyelitis has a mortality of approximately 80%

27 The following are true of MRI:
- a) On proton-density weighted images of the brain, the grey matter is brighter than the white matter
- b) Short inversion recovery (STIR) sequences have a short echo time
- c) Fluid attenuated inversion recovery is useful for identifying plaques adjacent to the ventricles
- d) Wide slice width requires a wide bandwidth
- e) The Larmor frequency is proportional to the gyromagnetic ratio

28 Concerning sellar masses:
- a) Craniopharyngioma is the commonest childhood sellar mass
- b) Craniopharyngioma is more commonly calcified in adults than children
- c) Craniopharyngioma usually contains bright areas on T1 weighted images
- d) Craniopharyngioma normally has a regular outline on imaging
- e) Rathke's cleft cyst develops from squamous epithelium in the sphenoid sinus

29 Regarding the leukodystrophies:
- a) Metachromic leukodystrophy is the commonest subtype
- b) Adrenoleukodystrophy is inherited in autosomal recessive fashion
- c) Leigh's disease affects the basal ganglia
- d) Metachromic leukodystrophy affects the basal ganglia
- e) Infants with Canavan's disease may have increased cranial circumference

30 Concerning assessment of the submandibular space:
- a) The vast majority of benign submandibular tumours are pleomorphic adenomas
- b) Adenocarcinoma is the commonest malignant submandibular tumour
- c) Pleomorphic adenomas are typically homogenous hyperechoic lesions on ultrasound
- d) Between 80-90% of salivary gland calculi occur in the submandibular space
- e) The earliest sign of Sjögren's disease on ultrasound is hypoechoic glandular enlargement

1 a) False - 300
b) True
c) True
d) True
e) True - elsewhere, malignant nodes tend to be round

Ying, Ahuja. Sonography of Neck Lymph Nodes - Part 1 Normal Nodes. *Clinical Radiology* 2003; 58: 351-8.

2 a) True
b) False - this is a branch of the basilar artery
c) True
d) False - basilar artery
e) False - basilar artery

Anatomy for Diagnostic Imaging. 2nd edition. Ryan, McNichols and Eustace. W.B. Saunders, 2004: 77-8.

3 a) True - usually middle-aged women
b) True - in 90%
c) False
d) False - this is seen with optic nerve sheath meningioma
e) False - unlike optic nerve sheath meningioma

Aids to Radiological Differential Diagnosis. 4th edition. Chapman and Nakielny. W.B. Saunders, 2003: 383.

4 a) True
b) False - 65-85%
c) True
d) False - fat-suppressed T2 weighted MRI in the axial plane
e) False - hypoechoic

Ahuja, *et al.* Imaging for Primary Hyperparathyroidism. *Clinical Radiology* 2004; 59: 967-76.

5 a) True - consisting of the caudate and lentiform nuclei
b) True
c) False
d) False
e) True

Anatomy for Diagnostic Imaging. 2nd edition. Ryan, McNichols and Eustace. W.B. Saunders, 2004: 55.

6 a) False - B-cell non-Hodgkin's lymphoma
b) True
c) False - hyperdense
d) False - intermediate to low signal on T2 weighted MRI due to high cell packing
e) True

Fundamentals of Diagnostic Radiology. 2nd edition. Brant and Helms. Lippincott, Williams and Wilkins, 1999: 125.

7 a) True
b) True
c) True
d) True
e) True

Aids to Radiological Differential Diagnosis. 4th edition. Chapman and Nakielny. W.B. Saunders, 2003: 391.

8 a) True
b) False - 80-85%
c) True - whereas cemento-ossifying fibroma may displace them or even resorb their roots
d) True
e) False - maxilla

Macdonald-jamkowski. Fibro-osseous Lesions of the Face and Jaws. *Clinical Radiology* 2004; 59: 11-25.

9 a) True
b) False - very poor or no enhancement
c) True - accounts for 50% of gliomas
d) False - 70% show calcification on CT. 100% show calcification pathologically. However, a calcified brain tumour is still more likely to be an astrocytoma
e) False - frontal lobes mostly

Fundamentals of Diagnostic Radiology. 2nd edition. Brant and Helms. Lippincott, Williams and Wilkins, 1999: 118-21.

10 a) True
b) True - medulloblastoma is the commonest
c) False - 20% calcify
d) False - most commonly affect the pons
e) True

Fundamentals of Diagnostic Radiology. 2nd edition. Brant and Helms. Lippincott, Williams and Wilkins, 1999: 121-4.

11 a) False - perpendicular
b) False - cervical
c) True
d) False - 80%
e) False - this is true for brain lesions but not for spinal cord lesions

Fundamentals of Diagnostic Radiology. 2nd edition. Brant and Helms. Lippincott, Williams and Wilkins, 1999: 169-80.

12 a) True
b) False - 85% of cases
c) True
d) False - both pathologies respond in a similar way
e) True

Aviv, Miszkiel. Orbital Imaging: Part 2 Intraorbital Pathology. *Clinical Radiology* 2005; 60: 288-307.

13 a) True
b) True
c) False - on MRI, due to multiple small tumour vessels
d) True
e) False - most commonly inferior to base of skull, close to jugular foramen

Radiology Review Manual. 5th edition. Dahnert. Lippincott, Williams and Wilkins, 2003: 389.

14 a) True
b) True - idiopathic supraclinoid carotid artery obliterative arteriopathy mostly seen in children
c) True
d) True - seen in red wine drinking alcoholics
e) True - in children with measles

Fundamentals of Diagnostic Radiology. 2nd edition. Brant and Helms. Lippincott, Williams and Wilkins, 1999: 169-80.

15 a) True
b) False
c) False
d) False - fast gradient-echo sequence used in diffusion imaging
e) False - 0.5 line pairs per mm

Physics for Medical Imaging. Farr, Allisy-Roberts. Bailliere Tindell, 1996: 215-50.

16 a) False - commonest cause in young adults. *Haemophilus influenzae* is commonest cause in children
b) True
c) True
d) True
e) True

Fundamentals of Diagnostic Radiology. 2nd edition. Brant and Helms. Lippincott, Williams and Wilkins, 1999: 159-61.

17 a) True
b) False - superior thyroid artery
c) True
d) True
e) True

Anatomy for Diagnostic Imaging. 2nd edition. Ryan, McNichols and Eustace. W.B. Saunders, 2004: 41-2.

18 a) True - due to atrophy of the temporal lobes
b) False - the pars compacta is thinned
c) True
d) True - causing characteristic heart-shaped enlargement of the frontal horns
e) False - Wilson's disease

Fundamentals of Diagnostic Radiology. 2nd edition. Brant and Helms. Lippincott, Williams and Wilkins, 1999: 183-4.

19 a) True - leading to hydrocephalus
b) False - iso- or hyperdense
c) True - affects atria of lateral ventricles in children
d) False - high signal on T2 weighted imaging
e) False - 10-20%

Fundamentals of Diagnostic Radiology. 2nd edition. Brant and Helms. Lippincott, Williams and Wilkins, 1999: 139-40.

20 a) True - as this will increase voxel size
b) True
c) False - narrow receiver bandwidth
d) True
e) False

Physics for Medical Imaging. Farr, Allisy-Roberts. Bailliere Tindell, 1996: 215-50.

21 a) True
b) False - males
c) False - seen in 90% of cases
d) True - due to vascularity there is risk of haemorrhage
e) True

Radiology Review Manual. 5th edition. Dahnert. Lippincott, Williams and Wilkins, 2003: 381.

22 a) False - lateral third is cartilaginous. Medial two thirds are bony
b) True
c) False - the tegmen tympani, an important bony landmark. Once this is eroded disease may spread to the middle cranial fossa
d) True
e) False - oval window niche

Ahuja, *et al.* CT Imaging of the Temporal Bone, Normal Anatomy. *Clinical Radiology* 2003; 58: 681-6

23 a) False - most common
b) True - ratio of 2:1
c) True
d) True - from cochlear portion in 15%
e) False - hyperintense. However, meningioma remains hypointense or isointense on T2 weighted imaging

Radiology Review Manual. 5th edition. Dahnert. Lippincott, Williams and Wilkins, 2003: 312-3.

24 a) True
b) True
c) False - hypoechoic. However metastatic nodes from papillary carcinoma of the thyroid tend to be hyperechoic
d) False - papillary and medullary carcinoma
e) True

Ahuja, Ying. Sonography of Neck Lymph Nodes; Part 2 - Abnormal nodes. *Clinical Radiology* 2003; 58: 359-66.

25 a) False - large posterior communicating artery seen in 6-40% of people
b) True
c) False - 3%
d) True
e) True

Anatomy for Diagnostic Imaging. 2nd edition. Ryan, McNichols and Eustace. W.B. Saunders, 2004: 78-9.

26 a) True
b) True
c) True
d) True
e) False - 20%

Fundamentals of Diagnostic Radiology. 2nd edition. Brant and Helms. Lippincott, Williams and Wilkins, 1999: 155-9.

27 a) True
b) True - less than 80ms
c) True
d) True
e) True

Physics for Medical Imaging. Farr, Allisy-Roberts. Bailliere Tindell, 1996: 215-50.

28 a) True
b) False - 80% are calcified in children, 40% are calcified in adults
c) True - due to proteinaceous debris
d) False - lobulated and irregular
e) False - squamous epithelial remnants of the anterior lobe of the pituitary gland

Fundamentals of Diagnostic Radiology. 2nd edition. Brant and Helms. Lippincott, Williams and Wilkins, 1999: 130-2.

29
a) True - these are inherited abnormalities of formation and maintenance of myelin. They are associated with gradual mental and motor deterioration in childhood. Metachromic leukodystrophy is autosomal recessive and diffusely affects the white matter tracts
b) False - sex-linked, therefore boys only affected
c) True
d) False
e) True - also seen in Alexander's disease

Fundamentals of Diagnostic Radiology. 2nd edition. Brant and Helms. Lippincott, Williams and Wilkins, 1999: 180-1.

30
a) True
b) False - adenoid cystic carcinoma is the commonest
c) False - homogenous hypoechoic lesions producing distal acoustic enhancement
d) True
e) False - hyperechoic glandular enlargement

Howlett, *et al.* Sonographic Assessment of the Submandibular Space. *Clinical Radiology* 2004; 59: 1070-8.